Workbook for

RADIOLOGY for the
Dental Professional

Workbook for

RADIOLOGY for the
Dental Professional

JEANINE J. STABULAS-SAVAGE, RDH, BS, MPH
Assistant Clinical Professor of Radiology
New York University
College of Dentistry
New York, New York

ELSEVIER

ELSEVIER

3251 Riverport Lane
St. Louis, Missouri 63043

WORKBOOK FOR RADIOLOGY FOR THE DENTAL
PROFESSIONAL, TENTH EDITION

ISBN: 978-0-323-47934-9

Notices

Practitioners and researchers must always rely on their own experience and knowledge in evaluating and using any information, methods, compounds, or experiments described herein. Because of rapid advances in the medical sciences, in particular, independent verification of diagnoses and drug dosages should be made. To the fullest extent of the law, no responsibility is assumed by Elsevier, authors, editors, or contributors for any injury and/or damage to persons or property as a matter of product liability, negligence or otherwise, or from any use or operation of any methods, products, instructions, or ideas contained in the material herein.

Content Strategist: Kristin Wilhelm
Content Development Specialist: Diane Chatman
Publishing Services Manager: Deepthi Unni
Senior Project Manager: Kamatchi Madhavan
Cover Designer: Muthukumaran Thangaraj

Printed in the United States of America

Last digit is the print number: 9   8   7   6   5   4

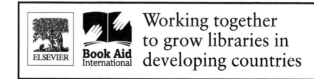

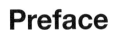

Preface

This study guide is intended to accompany the tenth edition of the textbook *Radiology for the Dental Professional.* The tenth edition of this workbook includes additional questions not included in the previous editions.

Each chapter in the workbook relates to a corresponding chapter in the textbook and stresses the essential information of the chapter through the use of definitions, short essays (comprehension), matching questions, completion, multiple choice, and ordering questions. The answers for the matching, completion, multiple choice, and ordering questions are available in the instructor's section of the Evolve resource site.

This edition also includes an entire section of activities that include illustrations designed to be utilized in a radiology workshop lab environment. This added feature can be used in a workshop lab or as an activity in the actual radiology lab when the student is not involved in simulated patient care.

Educational objectives are included at the beginning of each chapter to help the students focus on the material and concepts they are expected to learn and how this information is to be applied in the dental clinical setting.

The following suggestions will help students use this study guide to identify strengths and weaknesses.

1. Review the contents of each chapter before you attempt to do the exercise. Do not treat the questions individually and then refer to the text for the correct answer. Deal with the chapter's subject matter as a whole, since many of the questions are interrelated. This is a learning exercise meant to help you learn the material presented in the textbook, not an examination for grades.

2. Remember that the same subject matter may be repeated in different question forms in each chapter or other chapters, since the material overlaps. The subjects of the questions are not in the same order as they appear in the textbook, so don't expect to find a question in order for every page.

3. Read each question and study each illustration carefully in the Workshop Lab section before answering. You may know the answer or you may arrive at the correct answer by knowing which answers are incorrect.

This study guide is designed so that the pages can be easily removed, submitted if required, or placed in the student's notebook with the corresponding lecture notes.

Jeanine J. Stabulas-Savage

Contents

1 The History of Ionizing Radiation and Basic Principles of X-Ray Generation

EDUCATIONAL OBJECTIVES

After reading Chapter 1 of the textbook and completing this exercise, the student will be able to:
1. Define the key terms listed at the beginning of the chapter.
2. Recognize the names, dates, and discoveries of the early pioneers affiliated with the discovery and the use of x-radiation in dentistry.
3. Define the term *radiation* and distinguish it from the term and definition of *radioactive*.
4. Discuss *electromagnetic radiation* and the significance of the *electromagnetic spectrum*.
5. List and describe the properties of x-rays.
6. Identify and describe the components of an atom and the process of ionization.
7. List and describe each of the components and respective functions of the x-ray tube, and explain the significance of heat production in the x-ray tube.
8. Describe the production of x-rays in the x-ray tube.
9. Describe the interactions that could occur at the target of the anode, including general radiation (bremsstrahlung radiation) and characteristic radiation.

I. DEFINITIONS

Define/explain the following terms.

1. Anode _____

    _____

2. Atom _____

    _____

3. Bremsstrahlung (General) radiation _____

    _____

4. Cathode _____

    _____

5. Electromagnetic spectrum _____

    _____

6. Frequency _____

    _____

7. Hittorf-Crookes tube _____

    _____

8. Ionization _____

    _____

1

9. Nucleus _____

_____

10. Photons _____

_____

11. Radiation _____

_____

12. Radioactive _____

_____

13. Thermionic emission effect _____

_____

14. Wavelength _____

_____

15. X-rays _____

_____

II. COMPREHENSION EXERCISE

1. Explain the differences and similarities between radio waves and x-rays and their significance in dental radiology.

2. Explain why the dental x-ray machine is said to be "inefficient" in the production of x-radiation.

3. What is the source of the heat produced in the dental x-ray tube?

4. Explain the difference between duty rating and duty cycle.

5. Compare the binding energy of the various shells of an atom.

6. Clarify the difference between characteristic x-rays and Bremsstrahlung (General) x-rays.

7. Explain the function of the molybdenum focusing cup.

8. What accounts for ionizing radiation's potential to cause harmful biologic effects? Explain.

9. Cite the reasons for using tungsten as the material for the target in the dental x-ray tube.

10. Explain the difference between the filament and the high-tension circuit in the dental x-ray tube.

11. Describe the difference between the on/off switch and the exposure switch.

12. Compare the source of electrons in the original x-ray tubes with today's tubes.

13. List at least five properties of x-radiation as evidenced in dental radiographic procedures.

14. State the significance of the high-tension circuit in the production of x-rays in dentistry.

15. What is the relationship between the "wavelength" of a specific radiation and its ability to penetrate opaque structures?

4

III. MATCHING

Match the items in *Column A* with the appropriate items in *Column B*.

Column A

_____ 1. electrons
_____ 2. binding energy
_____ 3. focal spot
_____ 4. particulate radiation
_____ 5. Hittorf-Crookes tube
_____ 6. unit of x-ray exposure
_____ 7. 70 kV or above
_____ 8. protons
_____ 9. short wavelengths
_____ 10. ionization
_____ 11. focusing cup
_____ 12. unstable isotopes
_____ 13. thermionic emission effect
_____ 14. shells
_____ 15. atomic mass

Column B

a. fixed orbits
b. cathode
c. gamma rays
d. number of protons
e. electron cloud
f. anode
g. tungsten filament
h. negative charge
i. number of neutrons
j. beta particles
k. characteristic x-rays
l. positive charge
m. x-rays
n. K shell
o. Roentgen
p. roentgen
q. loss of an electron

IV. COMPLETE THESE STATEMENTS

1. An example of particulate radiation is

   _____,

   _____,

   _____,

   _____, or

   _____.

2. The effect of electromagnetic radiation on living organisms varies depending on the

   _____.

3. The amount of energy contained in electromagnetic radiation is determined by

   their _____ and

   _____.

4. Electric current within the dental x-ray tube flows

   from a _____ pole to a

   _____ pole.

5. Patients undergoing cancer therapy may receive radiation treatment from

   _____.

6. When atoms have the same atomic number but different atomic mass numbers, they are called

   _____.

7. A _____ is the smallest particle of a substance that retains the properties of the substance.

8. Individual units of radiation energy are referred

   to as _____.

9. In the dental x-ray machine the amount of energy produced at the anode as heat is

   _____%.

10. X-rays can affect a photographic emulsion that, when processed, produces

    _____.

11. The _____ refers to the number of consecutive seconds a machine can be operated before overheating.

12. Particulate radiations most commonly are emitted from radioactive substances called

_____.

13. Two examples of electromagnetic radiation

are _____ and

_____.

14. The three basic elements of an x-ray tube needed to produce x-rays are:

(1) _____ ,

(2) _____ , and

(3) _____ .

15. The milliamperage setting controls the

_____ of electrons that "boil off" the tungsten filament.

V. MULTIPLE CHOICE

Select the best answer.

1. Which of the following occurs at 70 kV or higher and accounts for a very small part of the x-rays produced in the dental x-ray machine?
   a. Bremsstrahlung radiation
   b. Compton scatter
   c. Characteristic radiation
   d. Coherent scatter
   e. Photoelectron interaction

2. Which of the following delineates where the thermionic emission effect takes place?
   a. tungsten target
   b. focal area
   c. tungsten filament of the anode
   d. tungsten filament of the cathode
   e. step-down transformer

3. The person accredited with the initial discovery of x-rays is
   a. Dr. Otto Walkhoff
   b. William D. Coolidge
   c. Wilhelm Conrad Roentgen
   d. Thomas Alva Edison
   e. Dr. C. Edmund Kells

4. You turn on the dental x-ray machine in the morning for your first patient. In doing so, you
   a. activate the high-tension circuit
   b. heat the anode
   c. activate the filament circuit
   d. turn on the step-up transformer
   e. produce x-rays

5. Which of the following electrons has the greatest binding energy?
   a. N shell electrons
   b. M shell electrons
   c. L shell electrons
   d. K shell electrons
   e. None of the above

6. X-rays are generated when a stream of electrons traveling from one side of a vacuum tube is stopped suddenly by its impact on the
   a. filament cup
   b. tungsten target of the anode
   c. tungsten target of the cathode
   d. focusing cup
   e. copper stem

7. Which of the following does not occur when the high voltage circuit is activated?
   a. The x-ray machine produces an audible and visible signal.
   b. Electrons travel from the filament to the target.
   c. Heat is produced.
   d. Electrons produced at the cathode fire across the tube and hit the target.
   e. X-rays are produced at the filament.

8. All of the following are examples of electromagnetic radiation *except*
   a. x-rays
   b. beta rays
   c. gamma rays
   d. microwaves
   e. light waves

9. Which of the following statements are *not* true concerning radioactive substances?
   a. They are utilized in cancer therapy.
   b. They are unstable elements.
   c. They produce high-energy waves.
   d. They are utilized to produce an image in dental radiography.
   e. All of the above are true.

10. Which of the following is incorrect?
    a. X-rays do not have a charge.
    b. X-rays do not have weight.
    c. X-rays travel at the speed of sound.
    d. X-rays have short wavelengths.
    e. X-rays cause ionization in tissues.

11. The dental x-ray tube is said to be "inefficient" because
    a. energy flows from the negative to the positive pole
    b. 1% of the energy produced is x-radiation
    c. the radiation produced is x-radiation
    d. it has a duty rating and a duty cycle
    e. it can overheat if used too frequently

12. As a result of the multiple Bremsstrahlung reactions,
    a. a heterogeneous x-ray spectrum is produced
    b. the succeeding x-rays produced will have less energy
    c. the later x-rays produced have less penetrating ability
    d. the wavelengths are different
    e. All of the above are valid statements.

13. Which of the following has the ability to affect living organisms?
    a. supervoltage x-rays
    b. microwaves
    c. magnetic resonance imaging
    d. electric waves
    e. ultrasonic waves

14. To prevent the x-ray tube and its components from overheating,
    a. each machine has a duty cycle and a duty rating
    b. the milliamperage setting should not exceed 15
    c. rotating anodes are utilized in extraoral radiography
    d. the copper sleeve surrounds the target
    e. All of the above are true.

15. The radiation produced at the atomic level in dental radiography is predominantly as a result of
    a. characteristic radiation
    b. radioactivity
    c. gamma rays
    d. Bremsstrahlung
    e. total energy loss

VI. TRUE/FALSE

Select whether each statement is true (**T**) or false (**F**). Circle the correct answer.

1. The focusing cup is found at the cathode. **T/F**
2. Bremsstrahlung radiation is the main source of radiation in the dental tube. **T/F**
3. X-rays are weightless. **T/F**
4. Ten percent of all reactions in the tube produce heat. **T/F**
5. X-rays are a type of ionizing radiation. **T/F**

VII. ORDERING QUESTIONS

Place the numbers 1, 2, 3, 4, and 5 in the spaces provided below to indicate the proper ordering sequence for the following questions.

1. Put the following pioneers and their discoveries in the order that they occurred from the earliest to the latest discovery:

    _____ Dr. Howard Riley Raper published the first Dental Radiology textbook.

    _____ William D. Coolidge invented the prototype of the contemporary x-ray tube.

    _____ Wilhelm Conrad Roentgen discovered the x-ray.

    _____ Dr. C. Edmund Kells took the first intraoral radiograph in the United States.

    _____ Dr. Otto Walkhoff is credited with the first dental use of the x-ray.

2. Put the following types of electromagnetic radiation in their proper order from the smallest to the longest wavelengths:

    _____ Dental radiography

    _____ Microwaves

    _____ Supervoltage x-rays

    _____ Ultraviolet rays

    _____ Television rays

3. Put the following functions of the dental x-ray tube in the order that they occur (from first to last):

    _____ X-rays are formed.

    _____ The tungsten filament heats up.

    _____ The cathode ray hits the tungsten target.

    _____ The electron cloud is formed.

    _____ The primary beam is filtered and collimated.

2 The Dental X-Ray Machine

EDUCATIONAL OBJECTIVES

After reading Chapter 2 of the textbook and completing this exercise, the student will be able to:

1. Define the key terms listed at the beginning of the chapter.
2. Discuss the following related to electricity:
   - Differentiate between an alternating current (AC) and direct current (DC) and their uses in the dental x-ray machine.
   - Explain what is meant by *rectification* in older dental x-ray units.
   - Know how many impulses there are in a second and how they are related to the exposure time settings in dental radiography.
   - Define *voltage*, and differentiate between kilovolt (kV) and kilovoltage peak (kVp).
   - Define *amperage*, and explain what the milliamperage (mA) setting controls in the dental x-ray machine.
   - Discuss the function of a transformer, and name the three transformers used in dental radiography, as well as their respective purposes.
   - Discuss the process of x-ray production in the dental x-ray tube, including the components, their functions, and the electrical system utilized.
3. Discuss the two major circuits in the x-ray machine.
4. Differentiate between older and newer dental x-ray machines, and discuss timers.
5. Describe the following related to x-ray beams:
   - Discuss the process of collimation of the x-ray beam and the role of the position-indicating device (PID) in this process.
   - Summarize the three parameters of the dental x-ray machine (quality, quantity, and exposure time) and how kV and mA are related to these parameters.
   - Define and apply the concept of a *half-value layer (HVL)* in describing the x-ray beam quality and penetration.
   - Discuss the significance of the intensity of the x-ray beam and how it is related to the quality, quantity, exposure time, and target-receptor distance (or focal-film distance [FFD]).
   - Discuss the significance and regulation of filtration and collimation as they apply to the dental x-ray beam.
   - Explain why rectangular collimation is considered to be an important factor in reducing radiation exposure to the dental patient.

I. DEFINITIONS

Define/explain the following terms.

1. Alternating current _____

_____

2. Central ray _____

_____

3. Collimation _____

_____

4. Direct current _____

_____

5. Electric current _____

_____

6. Filtration _____

_____

7. Half-value layer (HVL) _____

_____

8. Inherent filtration _____

_____

9. Rectangular collimation _____

_____

10. Rectification _____

_____

11. Scatter radiation _____

_____

12. Transformer _____

_____

13. Total filtration _____

_____

14. Useful beam _____

_____

15. Voltage _____

_____

II. COMPREHENSION EXERCISE

1. Explain the difference between filtration and collimation of the x-ray beam. What is the clinical significance of each?

2. Explain the difference between milliamperage and kilovoltage in the dental x-ray machine. What is the clinical significance of each?

3. Explain the concept of milliampere seconds (mAs).

4. Explain why exposure times are best expressed in impulses rather than in fractions of seconds.

5. What is rectangular collimation? Why is it important?

6. Do all x-ray photons at the anode of the x-ray tube have the same energy? Why? If not, what is done to correct this situation?

7. Explain why the use of an alternating current produces a heterogeneous x-ray beam.

8. What is the ideal size and shape of an intraoral x-ray beam?

9. What are the types of transformers used in the dental x-ray machine, and what is their function?

10. Why are electronic timers recommended for contemporary use as opposed to the utilization of the old mechanical timers?

11. What factors determine the intensity of the x-ray beam? Explain your answer.

12. Why is the half-value layer a more appropriate means of describing beam quality and penetration than kilovoltage?

13. What factors are used to determine the milliampere seconds required at a given kilovoltage? What is the clinical significance of using a higher milliamperage and a shorter exposure time?

14. What are the federal regulation specifications regarding total filtration of the x-ray beam at various kilovoltage settings?

15. Why would a change to rectangular collimation increase the incidence of collimator cutoff? How could this change be achieved without evidence of an increase in this exposure error?

III. MATCHING

Match the items in *Column A* with the appropriate items in *Column B.*

Column A

_____ 1. lead diaphragm
_____ 2. impulse
_____ 3. filtration
_____ 4. ampere
_____ 5. useful beam
_____ 6. rectangular collimation
_____ 7. electricity
_____ 8. quantity of x-rays
_____ 9. cycle
_____ 10. pointed cone
_____ 11. position-indicating device (PID)
_____ 12. rectification
_____ 13. half-value layer (HVL)
_____ 14. mechanical timers
_____ 15. quality of x-rays

Column B

a. removes long wavelengths
b. collimating device
c. x-ray beam after filtration and collimation
d. kilovoltage control
e. open-ended cylinder/rectangle
f. scatter radiation
g. x-ray beam penetration
h. energy source for radiation production
i. $\frac{1}{60}$ second margin of error
j. comparable to #2 size film packet
k. milliamperage control
l. lead
m. $\frac{1}{60}$ of a second
n. electrical current reversal blocking
o. x-rays
p. measures electrical current flow
q. flow and reversal of electrical current

IV. COMPLETE THESE STATEMENTS

1. The closed-end pointed cone should not be used as a

   PID because it creates _____.

2. The diameter of the x-ray beam for intraoral radiographs, measured at the face, should be no larger than

   _____.

3. Filtration of the dental x-ray beam is necessary because

   the beam contains _____,

   _____ x-rays.

4. In a dental x-ray machine operating at 75 kV, the required total filtration would be _____.

5. If the kilovoltage is increased with no other change in exposure factors, the resultant film will appear

   _____ and _____.

6. Limiting the size and shape of the x-ray beam is called

   _____.

7. On the control panel of the x-ray machine, the penetrating power of the x-ray beam is controlled by

   the _____ dial, and the number of x-rays produced is controlled by the

   _____ dial.

8. In real time, 20 impulses represent _____ second.

9. Limiting the size of the x-ray beam to just slightly larger than the actual size of the film packet is done

   by using _____.

10. Various dental x-ray machine models are designed to

    supply _____ rectification in which the portion of the alternating cycle is reversed.

11. The term _____ is used to denote the maximum voltage that is described by the sine wave that plots the alternation of the current.

12. Some dental x-ray machines have preset fixed milli-amperage choices, usually at _____, _____, or _____ mA.

13. The x-ray at the midpoint of the beam is known as the _____ ray.

14. Radiation protection codes in many states require the use of lead-lined, _____ PIDs.

15. The three parameters of the dental x-ray beam that are adjusted from the control panel are

    (1) _____,

    (2) _____,

    and (3) _____.

V. MULTIPLE CHOICE

Select the best answer.

1. Filters are used in the x-ray beam to
   a. increase density
   b. reduce density
   c. reduce exposure time
   d. correct the size of the beam
   e. reduce patient radiation dose

2. Proper collimation of the x-ray beam for film size and target-receptor (focal-film) distance will
   a. improve image definition
   b. increase radiographic contrast
   c. increase the intensity of the central beam
   d. increase secondary radiation
   e. reduce primary radiation

3. The best way to describe the penetration of an x-ray beam is by its
   a. half-value layer
   b. kilovoltage
   c. milliamperage
   d. rad output
   e. roentgen output

4. The milliampere control dial on the dental x-ray machine
   a. regulates the step-up transformer
   b. determines the penetration of the x-ray
   c. regulates the quality of the radiation
   d. regulates the quantity of the radiation
   e. regulates scatter radiation

5. You have taken a radiograph of a patient with a large skeletal build. The resulting image does not show the bone trabeculation well and appears to be underpenetrated. The adjustment that should be made for the retake is
   a. reduce the mA
   b. reduce the exposure time
   c. increase the kVp
   d. reduce the kVp
   e. check the processing solution temperature

6. In taking the radiograph, you did not center the beam on the receptor in the patient's mouth. The resulting image will show
   a. fogging
   b. overlapping
   c. elongation
   d. collimator cutoff (cone cutting)
   e. foreshortening

7. The dental x-ray machine in your office operates at 90 kV and thus is required to have a total filtration of
   a. 2.75 inches of aluminum
   b. 2.5 inches of aluminum
   c. 2.0 mm of aluminum
   d. 2.5 mm of aluminum
   e. 1.5 mm of aluminum

8. The radiation inspector comes to your office and tells you that your x-ray beam has an HVL of 1.00 mm of aluminum. You should
   a. feel assured that the beam meets the recommended standards
   b. be concerned because of the unnecessary secondary radiation to your patients
   c. be concerned because the beam is too penetrating
   d. add more filtration
   e. use a different PID

9. The x-ray beam from a conventional dental machine is
   a. a continuous beam
   b. a convergent beam
   c. a continuous divergent beam
   d. a pulsating divergent beam
   e. none of the above

10. Using a 16-inch target-receptor distance, the diameter of the beam measured at the patient's face should be no larger than
    a. 1 inch
    b. 3 inches
    c. 2.75 cm
    d. 1.5 cm
    e. 2.75 inches

11. For x-ray timers calibrated in impulses, how many impulses are there in a second?
    a. 10
    b. 30
    c. 60
    d. 120
    e. 15

12. The intensity of the beam is affected by the
    a. kilovolt peak
    b. milliamperage
    c. exposure time
    d. target-receptor (focal-film) distance
    e. all of the above

13. How many times per second is the polarity reversed in a dental x-ray machine operating on an alternating current?
    a. 30
    b. 15
    c. 60
    d. 45
    e. none of the above

14. The high-voltage circuit in the dental x-ray machine requires voltage in the range of 65,000 to 100,000, which is achieved by the use of the
    a. step-up transformer
    b. high-tension circuit
    c. autotransformer
    d. low-tension circuit
    e. step-down transformer

15. Which of the following materials is most resistant to x-radiation?
    a. copper
    b. molybdenum
    c. tungsten
    d. lead
    e. aluminum

VI. TRUE/FALSE

Select whether each statement is true (**T**) or false (**F**). Circle the correct answer.

1. Milliamperage determines the speed of the electrons. **T/F**
2. The dental x-ray tube is self-rectified. **T/F**
3. The dental x-ray beam is homogeneous. **T/F**
4. Kilovoltage determines the penetration of the beam. **T/F**
5. In a 60-cycle alternating current, there are 30 pulses of x-ray per second. **T/F**

VII. ORDERING QUESTIONS

Place the numbers 1, 2, 3, 4, and 5 in the spaces provided below to indicate the proper ordering sequence for the following questions.

1. Put the following occurrences that take place in regard to the initial phase of x-ray production in the order of their occurrence (from first to last):

    _____ The step-down transformer reduces 110 volts to 3-5 volts.

    _____ The tungsten filament heats up.

    _____ The x-ray machine is turned on and activates the filament circuit.

    _____ The thermionic emission effect occurs.

    _____ The electron cloud is formed.

2. Put the following occurrences that take place in regard to the secondary phase of x-ray production in the order of their occurrence (from first to last):

    _____ The electrons strike the tungsten target.

    _____ The exposure button is pressed and the high-voltage circuit is activated.

    _____ The molybdenum focusing cup directs the cathode ray toward the target of the anode.

    _____ The x-rays travel through the porte, aluminum filter, and collimators toward the patient.

    _____ The step-up transformer increased the 110 volts to 65,000-100,000 volts.

3. Put the following steps in x-ray production in the order that they occur (from first to last):

    _____ Primary radiation is formed.

    _____ The electrons are formed at the cathode.

    _____ The electrons strike the tungsten target.

    _____ Secondary (scatter) radiation is formed.

    _____ The useful beam leaves the x-ray tube head through the PID and strikes the patient.

3 Image Formation

EDUCATIONAL OBJECTIVES

After reading Chapter 3 of the textbook and completing this exercise, the student will be able to:

1. Define the key terms listed at the beginning of the chapter.
2. Discuss the following related to density and contrast:
   - Define *density* and *contrast.*
   - Know the differences between *short-scale contrast* and *long-scale contrast,* as well as the differences between *high contrast* and *low contrast,* and the kilovolt (kV) settings for each of these types of contrast.
   - List the determining factors of object contrast.
   - List the causes of film fog and its effect on image contrast.
3. Discuss the factors that will produce diagnostic radiographs in terms of image sharpness, resolution, detail, and definition. In addition:
   - Define and discuss the differences between the umbra and penumbra.
   - Explain what is meant by a *recessed tube* or *recessed target.*
   - Explain the significance of the inverse square law in dental radiography and know how to calculate the mathematical equations associated with this law.
4. List and describe the factors that will minimize image distortion and enlargement, as well as explain the effect that movement during an exposure can have on the resultant image.

I. DEFINITIONS

Define/explain the following terms.

1. Actual focal area _____

   _____

2. Bisecting-angle technique _____

   _____

3. Blurred image _____

   _____

4. Contrast _____

   _____

5. Detail _____

   _____

6. Effective focal area _____

   _____

7. Film density _____

   _____

8. Film fog _____

_____

9. Target-receptor distance (focal-film distance, FFD) _____

_____

10. Illuminator (viewbox) _____

_____

11. Image magnification _____

_____

12. Inverse square law _____

_____

13. Long-scale contrast _____

_____

14. Object density _____

_____

15. Object-receptor distance (object-film distance, OFD) _____

_____

16. Paralleling technique _____

_____

17. Penumbra _____

_____

18. Recessed tube (recessed target) _____

_____

19. Short-scale contrast _____

_____

20. Umbra _____

_____

II. COMPREHENSION EXERCISE

1. What factors determine film contrast?

2. What is the ideal technique and setting for viewing radiographs?

3. What is the importance of the target area size?

4. What are the factors that influence image detail?

5. What is the ideal relationship in intraoral radiography of the central ray, tooth, and receptor? Can this be achieved?

6. Does the patient receive a larger radiation dose with the longer exposures in the 16-inch FFD technique than with a comparable radiograph using the 8-inch FFD technique?

7. Explain how an increased FFD compensates for an increased OFD while using the paralleling radiographic exposure technique?

8. Why is there less image magnification with a 12-inch FFD than with an 8-inch FFD?

9. Name the possible types of movement that could occur in dental radiography and their respective consequences.

10. What are the advantages of using a 90-kV setting rather than a 65-kV setting?

11. Why is an FFD of greater than 16 inches not recommended?

12. What criteria must be met in terms of definition, image enlargement, and distortion to produce the "ideal radiograph" of a tooth or other structure?

13. What factors determine object contrast?

14. What would the result be of using an FFD of less than 8 inches?

15. What is meant by the concept of a recessed tube (recessed target)? What is its purpose?

16. Explain the difference between long-scale and short-scale film contrast. How are they determined?

17. When changing from an 8-inch FFD to a 16-inch FFD, what changes, if any, must be made to the collimator?

18. Explain the inverse square law. Give two clinical applications of its use.

19. What are the advantages of the 16-inch FFD technique over the 8-inch technique?

20. What is the ultimate goal of dental radiography regardless of the type of imaging system used?

III. MATCHING

Match the items in *Column A* with the appropriate items in *Column B*.

Column A

_____ 1. blurred image
_____ 2. tooth-receptor position
_____ 3. right-angle technique
_____ 4. long-scale contrast
_____ 5. inverse square law
_____ 6. penumbra
_____ 7. radiolucent
_____ 8. illuminator
_____ 9. focal area size
_____ 10. short-scale contrast
_____ 11. radiopaque
_____ 12. thin image
_____ 13. umbra
_____ 14. dense image
_____ 15. density

Column B

a. unsharpness
b. degree of blackness
c. high contrast
d. paralleling technique
e. x-ray intensity
f. viewbox
g. overexposed
h. white (light) areas
i. sharpness
j. object-receptor distance
k. patient movement
l. secondary radiation
m. underexposure
n. bisecting method
o. low contrast
p. black (dark) areas
q. detail

IV. COMPLETE THESE STATEMENTS

1. At present, most dental x-ray machines operate in the kV range of _____.

2. The size of the focal area at the anode in the dental x-ray machine influences greatly the _____ of the image.

3. The two types of related densities that are factors in image formation are the _____ and _____ densities.

4. The milliampere range for an intraoral x-ray machine is _____.

5. Image _____ is the visual quality of a radiograph that depends on definition or sharpness.

6. Using an aluminum step wedge, large gray areas occur when using a _____ -kV setting as compared with a 65-kV setting.

7. The difference in the degree of blackness between adjacent areas on a radiograph is the _____.

8. Two advantages of the 16-inch FFD over the 8-inch FFD are _____ and _____.

9. In a periapical radiograph, the milliamperage required for an exposure to produce an acceptable radiograph is determined mainly by the _____.

10. Many in the field of dental radiography believe that the human eye can detect changes better in the _____ -kV to _____ -kV range.

11. The main disadvantage of the bisecting technique for periapical radiography is _____.

12. The total energy in the x-ray beam in a specific area and at a given time is called the _____.

13. The actual focal area size is _____ than the effective focal area size in a dental x-ray tube.

14. The limiting factor on how small the focal area can be in the dental x-ray tube is the _____.

15. _____ is the term that describes the area of sharpness in an acceptable radiograph.

V. MULTIPLE CHOICE

Select the best answer.

1. A 16-inch cylinder is used in the paralleling technique to
   a. reduce secondary radiation
   b. avoid magnification of the image
   c. avoid distortion of the image
   d. avoid superimposition of anatomic structures
   e. facilitate correct vertical angulation of the position-indicating device (PID)

2. As the distance between the end of the PID and the receptor increases, the
   a. intensity of the x-ray beam decreases
   b. possibility of film fogging decreases
   c. density of the film image increases
   d. possibility of collimator cutoff decreases
   e. sharpness of the film is affected

3. Image sharpness on a radiograph is increased by
   a. using a large focal spot size
   b. using a small focal spot size
   c. increasing the OFD
   d. decreasing target skin distance
   e. increasing exposure time

4. You have decided to switch the PID in your office, replacing the 8-inch cylinder with a 16-inch cylinder. Using D-speed film, the milliamperage will remain the same, as will the kilovolt peak. The old exposure for lower premolars was 12 impulses; the new exposure to obtain images of equal density will be
   a. 40 impulses
   b. 30 impulses
   c. 20 impulses
   d. 1 second
   e. 48 impulses

5. As stated in the previous question, after changing to a 16-inch PID, you decide to change from D- to E-speed film. The new exposure at the same milliamperage and kilovolt peak for the lower premolar will be
   a. 80 impulses
   b. 24 impulses
   c. 10 impulses
   d. 1 second
   e. 30 impulses

6. The most likely cause for an image with very poor definition is
   a. a large focal area
   b. a very short FFD
   c. patient movement
   d. use of the bisecting technique
   e. use of the paralleling technique

7. A radiograph that has many dark and light areas but few gray areas is said to have
   a. high density
   b. low density
   c. high contrast
   d. low contrast
   e. none of the above

8. To increase contrast, the operator should decrease the
   a. exposure time
   b. milliamperage
   c. OFD
   d. film speed
   e. kilovolt peak

9. Use of a kilovolt peak between 45 and 65 produces
   a. scatter radiation
   b. fogging
   c. a blurred image
   d. an underexposed image
   e. none of the above

10. The difference in degrees of blackness on a radiograph is called
    a. density
    b. tone
    c. contrast
    d. fogging
    e. shades

11. A long FFD is desirable because
    a. more radiation is absorbed by the tissues
    b. the resulting radiation is more penetrating
    c. more soft radiation strikes the object
    d. the central rays of the primary beam are less divergent
    e. overexposure rarely occurs

21

12. Radiographs should always be viewed
    a. in a well-lit room
    b. on a viewbox
    c. in the operatory
    d. by holding them up to a ceiling light
    e. using light from a window

13. Which of the following materials is most effective in absorbing x-rays?
    a. gold
    b. composite
    c. enamel
    d. acrylic
    e. dentin

14. If the intensity of a beam of radiation is 12 at a point 12 inches from the target, the intensity of the beam at 24 inches is
    a. 2
    b. 3
    c. 4
    d. 5
    e. 6

15. You have taken a radiograph of a patient. The resulting image is thin (light). The adjustment that should be made for the retake is
    a. reduce the kilovolt peak
    b. reduce the exposure time
    c. increase the milliamperage
    d. reduce the milliamperage
    e. decrease the processing solution temperature

16. If the distance from the source of radiation to the receptor is decreased and no other adjustments are made, the resultant radiograph will
    a. be lighter
    b. be darker
    c. be more defined
    d. have an increased penumbra
    e. be unchanged

17. Changing from 75 kV to 90 kV will
    a. increase the radiolucency of the resultant radiograph
    b. decrease radiographic density
    c. decrease radiographic contrast
    d. increase radiographic contrast
    e. increase radiographic exposure time

18. Which of the following causes film fog on radiographs?
    a. underexposure
    b. scattered radiation
    c. improper safelighting
    d. light leak in the darkroom
    e. processing solutions that are too cold
       (1) a, b, c
       (2) a, b, c, d
       (3) a, b, e
       (4) b, c, d
       (5) b, c, d, e
       (6) c, d, e

19. If the PID is 2 inches away from the patient's skin instead of almost touching, the resulting radiograph will be
    a. underexposed
    b. overexposed
    c. overpenetrated
    d. foreshortened
    e. underpenetrated

20. The criteria for an acceptable radiograph include
    a. proper definition
    b. proper detail
    c. sharpness
    d. desirable contrast
    e. all of the above

VI. TRUE/FALSE

Select whether each statement is true (**T**) or false (**F**). Circle the correct answer.

1. The two types of related densities that are factors in image formation are the object density and the film density. **T/F**
2. Low-contrast films appear mainly black and white with very few gray tones. **T/F**
3. The smaller the focal area at the anode is, the better the image detail will be. **T/F**
4. The most common FFDs used in dentistry are 8, 12, and 20 inches. **T/F**
5. Image detail is not affected by movement. **T/F**

VII. ORDERING QUESTIONS

Place the numbers 1, 2, 3, 4, and 5 in the spaces provided below to indicate the proper ordering sequence for the following questions.

1. Put the following factors that influence object contrast in their ordered sequence from 1 to 5 as listed in Chapter 3 of the accompanying textbook:

   _____ Scatter radiation

   _____ The density of the object

   _____ The thickness of the object

   _____ The chemical composition of the object

   _____ The quality of the x-ray beam

2. Put the following mathematical steps in the proper order for calculating the change in time when the FFD is changed (from first to last):

   _____ Decide whether to multiply or divide the squared difference in distance with the original time.

   _____ Determine the difference in distance.

   _____ Square the difference in distance.

   _____ Compare the original distance with the new distance.

   _____ Remember if the distance is increased, the time increases and if the distance decreases, the time decreases.

3. Put the following 6 descriptions of contrast in order with their respective kV range below:

Long-scale contrast	High-contrast	Short-scale contrast
Black and white	Low-contrast	Shades of gray

   Low kV range =

   _____ = _____ = _____

   High kV range =

   _____ = _____ = _____

Image Receptors

EDUCATIONAL OBJECTIVES

After reading Chapter 4 of the textbook and completing this exercise, the student will be able to:
1. Define the key terms listed at the beginning of the chapter.
2. Discuss the evolution of the dental x-ray "packet" from 1896 until today.
3. Discuss the following related to film packets:
   ■ List the components of the film packet and the respective function of each component.
   ■ Discuss the composition of the film itself.
   ■ Define and describe the concepts of film speed and film sensitivity.
   ■ Explain what is meant by the term *film fog,* and discuss the sources of fogging.
4. Summarize the duplicating process in dental radiography.
5. Summarize the imaging system used in conventional extraoral radiography known as a *film-screen system.*
6. Differentiate between the sensors and the process utilized in direct versus indirect digital radiography.

I. DEFINITIONS

Define/explain the following terms.

1. ANSI film rating _____

   _____

2. Characteristic curve _____

   _____

3. Cassette _____

   _____

4. Direct digital imaging _____

   _____

5. Double-film packet _____

   _____

6. Extraoral projection _____

   _____

7. Film base _____

   _____

8. Film contrast _____

   _____

9. Film duplication _____

   _____

10. Film emulsion _____

    _____

11. Film reversal _____

_____

12. Film sensitivity _____

_____

13. Film-screen system _____

_____

14. Fluorescence _____

_____

15. Fog _____

_____

16. Indirect digital imaging _____

_____

17. Intensifying screen _____

_____

18. Orientation dot _____

_____

19. Phosphor _____

_____

20. Rare earth screen _____

_____

II. COMPREHENSION EXERCISE

1. What determines film speed? What film speed should be used?

2. Why should the dental professional consult the ANSI rating as opposed to the manufacturer's descriptive names when establishing the desired film speed for an exposure?

3. What special precautions must be taken in the darkroom when loading cassettes and processing extraoral film?

4. What are the advantages of using rare earth intensifying screens?

5. Explain the relationship between the size of the silver halide crystals and the detail/definition of the resulting radiograph.

6. List the direct digital sensors and indirect digital sensor used in digital imaging and state their main differences.

7. Explain the significance of film-screen compatibility.

8. How can the left side of the patient be differentiated from the right on extraoral and panoramic films?

9. How does the use of intensifying screens reduce the radiation needed to expose radiographs?

10. What is the purpose of the lead foil in the film packet?

11. Name the three main sources of film fog and briefly explain each.

12. Explain the difference between a double-emulsion film and a double-film packet.

13. How would you compare the milliampere seconds needed for E-speed film with that needed for F-speed film?

14. Describe the process of radiographic duplication.

15. How would you compare the radiation exposure to the patient using E-speed film with that using F-speed film?

16. What are silver halides? How are they used in dentistry?

17. What determines the speed of an intensifying screen?

18. List three uses for duplicate radiographs in dentistry.

19. Does the emulsion differ on a bitewing from the emulsion on a periapical film? If so, why?

20. Why should intensifying screens be used in extraoral radiography in spite of the loss of definition exhibited on the resultant radiographs?

III. MATCHING

Match the items in *Column A* with the appropriate items in *Column B*.

Column A

_____ 1. lead foil backing
_____ 2. pediatric film size
_____ 3. film fog
_____ 4. light fog
_____ 5. film density
_____ 6. single emulsion
_____ 7. flexible cassette
_____ 8. occlusal film
_____ 9. intensifying screen
_____ 10. F-speed film
_____ 11. green light
_____ 12. film duplication
_____ 13. orientation dot
_____ 14. film packet
_____ 15. chemical fog

Column B

a. large halide grains
b. gelatin
c. secondary radiation
d. #4 size
e. panoramic radiography
f. film mounting
g. decreased patient exposure
h. processing solutions
i. third-party payers
j. overall gray appearance
k. film emulsion
l. light leak
m. #0 size
n. rare earth intensifying screens
o. degree of blackness
p. duplicating film
q. light-tight

IV. COMPLETE THESE STATEMENTS

1. At present the ANSI dental film group that gives the patient the least amount of radiation exposure is _____.

2. The _____ presently used in dentistry are film, electronic digital sensors, and film-screen combinations.

3. In the early days of dental radiography, the x-ray _____ consisted of glass photographic plates or film cut into pieces and wrapped in black paper or rubber dam.

4. Long bitewing film packets are considered to be size # _____.

5. The plot for dental x-ray film that expresses the relationship between density of the film and the log relative exposure is the _____.

6. Extraoral films are processed in the _____ as intraoral films.

7. The main advantage in using rare earth intensifying screens is _____.

8. F-speed film will reduce radiation exposure by _____% when compared to D-speed film.

9. When comparing radiographic detail, it can be said that film-screen combinations produce _____ _____ detail when compared to film alone.

10. The component of an x-ray film described as a thin transparent coating that is placed over the emulsion is called the _____.

11. Duplicating film has a _____ emulsion.

12. Duplicating film has the emulsion on the _____ side of the film.

13. Double packets require slightly _____ exposure than single films.

14. It is said that the _____ the silver halide crystals are, the faster the speed of the film.

V. MULTIPLE CHOICE

Select the best answer.

1. When comparing ANSI film rated E with ANSI film rated F, one can say that
   a. F film is less sensitive
   b. F film requires more radiation
   c. F film results in more exposure to the patient
   d. F film requires less exposure time
   e. none of the above

2. Rare earth intensifying screens produce
   a. blue light
   b. red light
   c. green light
   d. ultraviolet light
   e. purple light

3. The best way to clean the intensifying screens in extra-oral cassettes is with
   a. detergent
   b. disinfectant solution
   c. cold sterilizing solution
   d. soapy water
   e. a wire brush

4. Film fog occurs when all or part of a radiograph is darkened by
   a. an imbalance or exhaustion of processing solutions
   b. a light leak
   c. improper safelighting
   d. scatter radiation
   e. All of the above are potential sources.

5. Which of the following statements is false concerning film duplication?
   a. The films to be duplicated are in close contact with the duplicating film.
   b. The shiny side of the film is the nonemulsion side.
   c. If less film density is needed on the duplicate radiograph, the exposure time is shortened.
   d. The raised portion of the orientation dot faces toward the light source.
   e. The radiographs being duplicated should be removed from their respective mounts.

6. Flexible cassettes are
   a. not used because of cracking of the emulsion
   b. used in all panoramic units
   c. used in some panoramic units
   d. used for lateral oblique projections only
   e. none of the above

7. Intraoral film packets must be
   a. resistant to salivary seepage
   b. flexible
   c. light-tight
   d. easy to open in the darkroom
   e. all of the above

8. To what does the term *film speed* refer?
   a. the developing time needed
   b. sensitivity to x-radiation
   c. half-life
   d. degree of blackness on the exposed radiograph
   e. shelf life

9. The advantage of a film that has emulsion on both sides is that
   a. the film requires less radiation exposure
   b. the image produced is less distorted
   c. the film has less sensitivity to radiation
   d. processing solutions work better
   e. the film is easier to mount

10. Which of the following film sizes is considered to be standard adult film?
    a. size #0
    b. size #1
    c. size #2
    d. size #3
    e. size #4

11. The intensifying screen that emits blue light and must be used with film that is sensitive to blue light is a
    a. nonlight screen
    b. calcium tungstate screen
    c. rare tungstate screen
    d. rare earth screen
    e. phosphor calcium screen

12. The device that converts x-ray energy into visible light is called a(n)
    a. cassette holder
    b. step-down transformer
    c. intensifying screen
    d. nonscreen film
    e. screen film

13. If the intensifying screens are not in perfect contact with the film, which of the following will occur?
    a. The screen may be damaged.
    b. The film may be damaged.
    c. There will be a light leak.
    d. There will be a loss of image sharpness.
    e. A thin film will result.

14. What is the major advantage in using the fastest speed film and high kilovolt peak?
    a. It increases film density.
    b. It increases film contrast.
    c. It produces a clearer image.
    d. It reduces the radiation exposure to the patient.
    e. It makes film easier and faster to develop.

15. The types of direct digital sensors that are used to produce an instantaneous image in digital imaging are
    a. APS sensors
    b. CCD sensors
    c. PSP plates
    d. CMOS sensors
    e. All of the above except "c" are correct answers.

VI. TRUE/FALSE

Select whether each statement is true (**T**) or false (**F**). Circle the correct answer.

1. The orientation dot on the film packet is useful in mounting. **T/F**
2. The lead foil in the film packet prevents collimator cut-off. **T/F**
3. The use of intensifying screens decreases exposure time. **T/F**
4. Pediatric film is size #3. **T/F**
5. D-speed film is currently recommended for use in dental radiography. **T/F**

VII. ORDERING QUESTIONS

Place the numbers 1, 2, 3, 4, and 5 in the spaces provided below to indicate the proper ordering sequence for the following questions.

1. Put the following steps in the evolution of dental film packets in the order that they happened from the earliest to the latest occurrence:

    _____ Kodak introduced the first commercially available prepackaged dental x-ray film.

    _____ Dental radiographic films are faster, reduce radiation exposure, and produce improved diagnostic images.

    _____ Kodak produced dental film packets in two speeds.

    _____ The x-ray packet consisted of glass photographic plates hand-wrapped in black paper or rubber.

    _____ Films were produced with double-coated (double-sided) emulsion.

2. Put the following components of a dental x-ray film packet in the order that they appear from the outside to the inside of the packet:

    _____ The x-ray film

    _____ The barrier envelope

    _____ The black paper film wrapper

    _____ The vinyl package wrapper

    _____ The lead foil backing

3. Put the following steps in duplicating radiographs in the order of their occurrence from the first to the last step:

    _____ Place the films to be duplicated in close contact with the duplicating film.

    _____ Process the duplicating film.

    _____ Set the timer on the duplicating machine.

    _____ Place the duplicating film with the emulsion side toward the light source.

    _____ Turn the white light off and the safelight on in the darkroom.

Biologic Effects of Radiation

EDUCATIONAL OBJECTIVES

After reading Chapter 5 of the textbook and completing this exercise, the student will be able to:
1. Define the key terms listed at the beginning of the chapter.
2. Describe the historical concern about the effects of ionizing radiation.
3. Discuss the ways in which x-rays interact with matter and the difference between direct and indirect effects of radiation.
4. Explain the difference between the definitions of exposure and dose and the units of radiation measurement for both, including their respective International System of Units (SI) conversions.
5. Define the basic terms and concepts related to the biologic effects of ionizing radiation on human tissue.
6. Discuss the factors that are related to a particular human tissue's sensitivity to radiation exposure. Also, define and give examples of *background radiation*.

I. DEFINITIONS

Define/explain the following terms.

1. Acute effects _____

_____

2. ALARA principle _____

_____

3. Background radiation _____

_____

4. Cell recovery _____

_____

5. Chronic effects _____

_____

6. Critical organs _____

_____

7. Deterministic or nonstochastic effects _____

_____

8. Dose equivalent _____

_____

9. Erythema dose _____

_____

10. Exposure _____

_____

11. Genetic cells _____

_____

12. Indirect effects of radiation _____

_____

13. Latent period _____

_____

14. Primary radiation _____

_____

15. Radiation caries _____

_____

16. Radiobiology _____

_____

17. Radioresistant _____

_____

18. Radiosensitive _____

_____

19. Somatic cells _____

_____

20. Stochastic effects _____

_____

II. COMPREHENSION EXERCISE

1. Explain the difference between radiation exposure and radiation dose.

2. What news events have created public concern of radiation exposure? What can dental professionals do to allay the fears associated with these occurrences?

3. What is the difference between a roentgen, a rad, and a rem?

4. What is the output of an x-ray machine? How is it measured?

5. Explain why the walls of the dental operatory do not become radioactive after continuous exposure to radiation.

6. Explain the difference between a localized dose and a total body dose.

7. What body cells are the most sensitive to ionizing radiation?

8. What is the difference between stochastic and deterministic or nonstochastic effects? Explain.

9. What is the primary mechanism for tissue change resulting from dental x-ray exposure?

10. What is the difference between a tissue that is radiosensitive and a tissue that is radioresistant? Explain.

11. How much background radiation does the population at sea level receive each year? What are the major sources of background radiation?

12. How does one handle the dental radiographic needs of a pregnant patient?

13. What are mutations? What can cause mutations in offspring?

14. Name some risks encountered in everyday living that compare with the risks of developing cancer from dental radiation.

15. Explain the risk vs. benefit concept.

16. What is the difference between primary and secondary radiation?

17. What is the erythema dose for facial skin? Is this an important consideration in dental radiology?

18. What does the latent period refer to in dental radiology?

19. What are the units for measuring radiation based on the metric system? How do these units relate to the conventional system?

20. Explain the difference between the acute and chronic effects of radiation.

III. MATCHING

Match the items in *Column A* with the appropriate items in *Column B*.

Column A

_____ 1. photoelectric effect

_____ 2. rad

_____ 3. total body exposure

_____ 4. ionization

_____ 5. acute effects of radiation

_____ 6. sievert

_____ 7. indirect effects of radiation

_____ 8. attenuation

_____ 9. dose equivalent

_____ 10. leukemia risk

_____ 11. Thompson scatter

_____ 12. roentgen

_____ 13. Compton effect

_____ 14. cell recovery

_____ 15. radiation therapy

Column B

a. free radical formation

b. happens 30% of the time

c. reduced x-ray beam intensity

d. more than 100 rads

e. coherent scatter

f. nuclear accident

g. 100 erg/g

h. cells' repair process

i. low-level radiation

j. radiation caries

k. happens 62% of the time

l. 100 rem

m. qualifying factor

n. free radicals

o. 1 esu/cc of air

p. kilovoltage

q. absorption of x-rays

IV. COMPLETE THESE STATEMENTS

1. The type of interaction between an x-ray photon and a loosely bound orbital electron is characterized by the _____ effect.

2. A pregnant woman in her sixth month can have, if deemed necessary, _____.

3. Radiation from medicine and dentistry accounts for about _____% of the average annual dose equivalent to the U.S. population.

4. The tissue most sensitive to ionizing radiation is _____.

5. Cellular changes caused by ionizing radiation are not passed on to succeeding generations in _____ tissue.

6. Our objective for the dental radiographic patient is to use the least amount of radiation to obtain _____.

7. The rate at which exposure to ionizing radiation occurs is called the _____.

8. The major component of background radiation at sea level is _____.

9. The objective for occupational radiation exposure is to keep the exposure as close to _____ as possible.

10. The time that elapses between the exposure to ionizing radiation and the appearance of clinical symptoms is called the _____.

11. In considering dental radiology, the roentgen, the rad, and the rem are _____.

12. One gray of radiation is equal to _____ rads.

37

13. An average skin exposure to the patient's face using E-speed film for a full-mouth series is about

_____.

14. The two mechanisms for tissue damage resulting from radiation exposure are _____

and _____ formation.

15. An example of an energy wave that will not cause

ionization is _____ or

_____.

16. An exposure of radiation is measured in _____.

17. The dose-response curve for dental radiation is a

_____.

18. An _____ placed in front of a dental x-ray machine's position-indicating device (PID) can indicate how many roentgens the machine is producing per second.

19. The occupational hazard for the pregnant dental professional under proper conditions should be

_____.

20. The greatest somatic hazard to patients from dental

x-rays is _____.

V. MULTIPLE CHOICE

Select the best answer.

1. In taking dental radiographs, the greatest dose of radiation to structures in the patient's jaw comes from
   a. the primary beam
   b. leakage from the x-ray machine
   c. scatter from the patient's face
   d. scatter from the PID
   e. secondary radiation

2. Ionization has occurred when
   a. cell death occurs
   b. photons penetrate matter
   c. radiant energy is converted to heat
   d. an electron is displaced from its orbit
   e. none of the above

3. Which form of radiation can cause ionization of atoms?
   a. radar
   b. microwaves
   c. radio waves
   d. visible light
   e. gamma rays

4. The ALARA principle refers to
   a. obtaining informed consent
   b. the disinfection procedures recommended in dental radiography
   c. obtaining diagnostically acceptable radiographs with minimal exposure to radiation
   d. decreasing the processing time for exposed radiographs
   e. none of the above

5. Patient radiation dose is related to which of the following?
   a. length of the exposure
   b. distance from the source
   c. shielding and filtration
   d. time of day
   e. position of the operator
      (1) a, b
      (2) a, b, c
      (3) a, b, c, d
      (4) a, c
      (5) none of the above

6. Which of the following travel at the greatest speed?
   a. x-rays
   b. gamma rays
   c. light
   d. microwaves
   e. They all travel at the same speed.

7. X-rays that are most likely to be absorbed by the skin are
   a. those with a short wavelength
   b. aluminum filtered rays
   c. those with long wavelengths
   d. high-energy waves
   e. sonic waves

8. Which of the following statements concerning background radiation is most accurate?
   a. It gives us the maximum recommended dosage for radiation exposure.
   b. It can be avoided if an individual is cautious.
   c. It is found everywhere.
   d. It is present only in dental offices and medical facilities.
   e. None of the above are correct.

9. Arrange the following cells and tissues from most sensitive to least sensitive to ionizing radiation.
   a. nerve
   b. bone
   c. lymphocytes
   d. gastrointestinal tract
      (1) b, a, d, c
      (2) c, a, d, b
      (3) c, b, a, d
      (4) c, d, a, b
      (5) c, d, b, a

10. In recent years the focus of prime concern from the effects of ionizing radiation used in dentistry has centered on
    a. somatic damage to the patient
    b. occupational exposure of dental workers
    c. genetic damage to patients
    d. cancer induction in patients
    e. its contribution to background radiation

11. Under the new metric system for measuring dose (SI), the rem is replaced by the
    a. rad
    b. gray
    c. sievert
    d. becquerel
    e. curie

12. Which of the following types of scatter radiation occurs most often with dental x-rays?
    a. Thompson
    b. Compton
    c. photoelectric
    d. coherent
    e. All of the above occur equally with dental x-rays.

13. The time period between exposure to x-rays and appearance of radiation damage is the
    a. silent period
    b. latent period
    c. waiting period
    d. refractory period
    e. gestation period

14. The Compton effect describes
    a. one type of interaction of x-rays with matter
    b. cell death
    c. cell recovery
    d. cell aberration
    e. cancerous change

15. The ALARA concept means
    a. always lower amperage requirements with age
    b. as low as reasonably achievable
    c. as low as recording allows
    d. as level as reasonably achievable
    e. none of the above

16. An angstrom unit is used to measure
    a. radiation dose
    b. radiation exposure
    c. x-ray wavelength
    d. half-value layer
    e. amperage

17. Which of the following statements are correct?
    a. X-rays can affect all living biologic tissue.
    b. Developing young immature cells are more sensitive to radiation.
    c. In dentistry only the primary beam is of concern for safety.
    d. Changes in adult cells are of short duration and are soon dissipated.
       (1) b, c, d
       (2) a, b, c
       (3) a, c, d, b
       (4) a, b

18. The unit that describes the amount of x-ray exposure in air is the
    a. rad
    b. rem
    c. roentgen
    d. gray
    e. sievert

19. The prime concern for dental personnel taking radiographs under accepted procedures is
    a. primary radiation
    b. secondary radiation
    c. Bremsstrahlung radiation
    d. classical radiation
    e. all of the above

20. Which of the following characteristics of body tissue determines its sensitivity to radiation?
    a. blood flow
    b. iron content
    c. oxyhemoglobin concentration
    d. mitotic rate
    e. water content

VI. TRUE/FALSE

Select whether each statement is true (**T**) or false (**F**). Circle the correct answer.

1. Secondary radiation is the radiation that comes directly from the dental x-ray tube. **T/F**
2. A free radical is an uncharged molecule and is initially very unstable. **T/F**
3. Dose is the amount of ionization in the air produced by x-rays. **T/F**
4. Background radiation can only occur naturally in the environment. **T/F**
5. The reproductive cells are not very radiosensitive. **T/F**

VII. ORDERING QUESTIONS

Place the numbers 1, 2, 3, 4, and 5 in the spaces provided below to indicate the proper ordering sequence for the following questions.

1. Put the following stages of the biologic effects of radiation in the order that they occur from the first to the last occurrence:

_____ Period of injury

_____ Cell recovery

_____ Radiation exposure

_____ Latent period

_____ Appearance of clinical symptoms

2. Put the following steps in taking a dental radiograph and the effects on the patient's body in the order they occur from the first to the last occurrence:

_____ A radiograph is taken.

_____ Radiation is absorbed by the skin, teeth, and bones.

_____ Other tissues absorb scatter radiation.

_____ Not all of the radiation reaches the receptor.

_____ Some radiation penetrates beyond the receptor.

3. Put the following human tissues in their respective category of radiosensitivity below:

Salivary glands
Growing bone
Bone marrow
Skin
Optic lens
Neurons
Lymphoid organs
Fine vasculature
Growing cartilage

High Radiosensitivity	Intermediate Radiosensitivity	Low Radiosensitivity
1. _____	1. _____	1. _____
2. _____	2. _____	2. _____
3. _____	3. _____	3. _____

6 Patient Protection

EDUCATIONAL OBJECTIVES

After reading Chapter 6 of the textbook and completing this exercise, the student will be able to:

1. Define the key terms listed at the beginning of the chapter.
2. Discuss patient protection and the ALARA principle (concept), as well as the role of the dental x-ray equipment in reducing radiation exposure to the patient before, during, and after the dental images are taken.
3. Describe the role of careful chairside techniques, processing techniques (when applicable), and image retrieval in reducing radiation exposure to the patient.
4. Define and recite the significance of radiation history, selection criteria, and the avoidance of administrative radiographs in patient protection.

I. DEFINITIONS

Define/explain the following terms.

1. Administrative radiographs _____

_____

2. ALARA principle (ALARA concept) _____

_____

3. Collimation _____

_____

4. Filtration _____

_____

5. Head leakage _____

_____

6. Lead apron _____

_____

7. Localizing ring _____

_____

8. Primary radiation _____

_____

9. Radiation history _____

_____

10. Retakes _____

_____

11. Secondary radiation _____

_____

12. Selection criteria _____

_____

13. Thyroid collar _____

_____

14. Tube head drift _____

_____

15. Useful beam _____

_____

II. COMPREHENSION EXERCISE

1. What was the problem with mechanical timers in dental x-ray machines? Explain.

2. Explain the effect of kilovoltage on patient dosage.

3. Why is the use of closed-ended pointed cones contraindicated in contemporary dentistry?

4. What is the advantage of using F-speed film and digital sensors in dental imaging? Explain.

5. Why is the paralleling technique preferred over the bisecting technique in regard to patient dosage?

6. What is the relationship between target-receptor distance (or focal-film distance, FFD) and patient dosage?

7. Define and give some examples of selection criteria for taking radiographs.

8. Why does a technique that employs overexposure with underdevelopment subject the patient to unnecessary radiation? Explain.

9. What is the present status of administrative radiographs?

10. List six major ways to reduce x-ray exposure for patients.

III. MATCHING

Match the items in Column A with the appropriate items in Column B.

Column A

_____ 1. postoperative radiographs
_____ 2. selection criteria
_____ 3. administrative radiographs
_____ 4. paralleling technique
_____ 5. increased FFD
_____ 6. change from E- to F-speed film
_____ 7. radiation history
_____ 8. mechanical timers
_____ 9. filtration
_____ 10. lead apron

Column B

a. decreased exit dose
b. remove soft wavelengths
c. medical/dental diagnostic and therapeutic radiation
d. root tip retrieval
e. reduce dose by 20%
f. not to be taken
g. inaccurate by ¼ of a second
h. required in many localities
i. inaccurate by a second
j. decreased thyroid dose
k. determines x-rays that are needed
l. 2¾-inch beam diameter

IV. COMPLETE THESE STATEMENTS

1. In an adult patient not prone to caries and clinically negative, bitewing radiographs should be taken every

   _____.

2. All new edentulous patients should _____.

3. Radiographs should always be viewed _____.

4. Taking radiographs to confirm the fit of restorations

   should be _____.

5. Retaking radiographs because of poor technique re-

   sults in _____.

6. _____ is the single most effective factor in reducing radiation exposure to the patient.

7. The thyroid dose in the bisecting method is greater

   because of _____.

8. The use of F-speed film will _____.

9. Mechanical timers are _____.

10. Kilovoltage of less than 65 should never be used for

    dental x-rays because _____.

V. MULTIPLE CHOICE

Select the best answer.

1. Using an F-speed rather than an E-speed film to produce a radiograph results in
   a. greater patient exposure
   b. less patient exposure
   c. the same exposure time
   d. a longer processing time
   e. a shorter processing time

2. All of the following reduce radiation exposure to the
   patient *except*
   a. rectangular collimation
   b. fast-speed film
   c. overexposure with underdevelopment
   d. lead aprons
   e. aluminum filtration

3. Which of the following combinations of dose reduction methods is most effective for reducing radiation
   for patients?
   a. F-speed film, round collimation
   b. F-speed film, lead apron
   c. F-speed film, rectangular collimation
   d. digital radiography, rectangular collimation
   e. digital radiography, lead apron

4. A dental x-ray machine operating at 75 kV is required to have a total aluminum filtration of
   a. 2 mm
   b. 2.5 mm
   c. 2 inches
   d. 2.5 inches
   e. 2.75 inches

5. Every radiographic retake represents
   a. an impulse of additional exposure to the patient
   b. a quadrupling of exposure to the patient
   c. an unnecessary doubling of patient exposure
   d. an attempt to improve one's technique without cost to the patient
   e. None of the above are relevant.

6. Which of these position-indicating devices (PIDs) is least effective in minimizing radiation scatter?
   a. lead-lined cylinder
   b. pointed cone
   c. lead-lined rectangle
   d. plastic cylinder
   e. plastic rectangle

7. Radiation history should include all of the following *except*
   a. medical radiation exposure
   b. dental radiation exposure
   c. therapeutic radiation exposure
   d. background radiation exposure
   e. panoramic radiation exposure

8. Lead aprons should be used
   a. on all patients
   b. to reassure patients
   c. to reduce scatter to the film
   d. only on children
   e. only on pregnant patients

9. All but which of the following are important to minimize patient exposure to radiation?
   a. proper collimation
   b. utilizing selection criteria to prescribe radiographs
   c. proper filtration
   d. darkroom quality assurance programs
   e. not repairing tube head drift

10. Dental radiographs should be taken
    a. only if there is pain
    b. to train students
    c. for insurance company requests
    d. routinely every 6 months
    e. to aid in diagnosis

11. Which of the following results in the greatest reduction to radiation in the patient?
    a. routine radiographs
    b. low kilovoltage peak
    c. digital sensors
    d. wide primary beam
    e. high milliamperage

12. According to selection criteria
    a. an asymptomatic edentulous patient does not require radiographs
    b. a 14-year-old patient will probably need posterior bitewings
    c. a panoramic exam is needed for a new edentulous patient
    d. very few patients need radiographs at 6-month intervals
    e. All of the above are correct.

13. The maximum diameter of the dental x-ray beam measured at the skin should be no greater than
    a. 2 mm
    b. 2.75 inches
    c. 2 inches
    d. 2.5 inches
    e. 2.75 mm

14. Before prescribing dental radiographs, which of the following are needed?
    a. history of previous radiographs
    b. clinical examination
    c. medical history
    d. dental history
    e. all of the above

15. The most important use of x-rays in dentistry is
    a. patient education
    b. legal protection
    c. diagnosis
    d. pain control
    e. therapy

VI. TRUE/FALSE

Select whether each statement is true (**T**) or false (**F**). Circle the correct answer.

1. The ALARA principle deals with radiation protection of the patient and operator. **T/F**
2. Pregnant patients may have radiographs taken when they are needed. **T/F**
3. The closed-ended pointed PID is recommended for use in dental radiography. **T/F**
4. Administrative radiographs should be strongly discouraged. **T/F**
5. The dose to the thyroid gland is greater in the bisecting angle technique. **T/F**

VII. ORDERING QUESTIONS

Place the numbers 1, 2, 3, 4, and 5 in the spaces provided below to indicate the proper ordering sequence for the following questions.

1. Put the following steps in "prescribing" dental radiographs for a particular patient in the order that they occur (from first to last):

    _____Selection criteria aid the dentist in choosing the radiographs.

    _____The patient is seated in the dental chair.

    _____The dental professional looks in the patient's mouth to determine the patient's risk for dental disease.

    _____The dental professional asks the patient questions regarding his or her radiation history.

    _____The ultimate decision is determined by the dentist's professional judgment.

2. Put the following equipment and techniques in their respective group regarding radiation protection for the dental patient:

Tube head drift
Skin exposure less than 2¾
Electronic timers
Receptor-holding devices
Head leakage
Rectangular collimation
kV below the acceptable range
Mechanical timers
Intensifying screens
Administrative radiographs
Bisecting technique
Lead aprons

Reduces radiation exposure to the patient

1. _____
2. _____
3. _____
4. _____
5. _____
6. _____

Increases radiation exposure to the patient

1. _____
2. _____
3. _____
4. _____
5. _____
6. _____

3. Put the following steps in x-ray exposure in the order that they occur in dental radiography (from first to last):

    _____ Scatter radiation

    _____ Primary radiation

    _____ Useful beam

    _____ Secondary radiation

    _____ Cathode ray

7 Operator Protection

EDUCATIONAL OBJECTIVES

After reading Chapter 7 of the textbook and completing this exercise, the student will be able to:
1. Define the key terms listed at the beginning of the chapter.
2. Discuss concepts related to operator dosage and protection, including maximum permissible dose (MPD), exposure technique, radiation monitoring, protective barriers, and the ALARA principle (concept).
3. Discuss how to deal with patients' concerns about and possible fear of dental radiographs.

I. DEFINITIONS

Define/explain the following terms.

1. Cumulative effective dose (CUMEfd) _____

   _____

2. Exposure technique _____

   _____

3. Film badge _____

   _____

4. Ionizing chamber _____

   _____

5. Maximum permissible dose (MPD) _____

   _____

6. Monitoring device _____

   _____

7. Pocket dosimeter _____

   _____

8. Protective barrier _____

   _____

9. Radiation monitoring _____

   _____

10. Radiation survey _____

   _____

II. COMPREHENSION EXERCISE

1. What does the acronym "CRESO" represent, and how does it apply to operator protection?

2. Where should the operator be positioned when taking radiographs?

3. Explain the significance of the present levels of the MPD.

4. What are the sources of potential radiation exposure to the radiographer?

5. What constitutes adequate shielding in the dental office? Are lead-lined walls always necessary?

6. What is the equation for determining the accumulated lifetime dose for a dental radiographer? What would it be for a 35-year-old?

7. What are the advantages of personnel wearing film badges over a radiation survey?

8. What should the operator "not do" in order to avoid primary beam exposure during a dental radiographic procedure?

9. Can dental workers continue to take radiographs during pregnancy? Explain.

10. List the ways the operator's occupational dose can be kept to zero.

III. MATCHING

Match the items in *Column A* with the appropriate items in *Column B*.

Column A

_____ 1. occupational MPD
_____ 2. nonoccupational MPD
_____ 3. maximum scatter
_____ 4. film badge
_____ 5. monitoring device
_____ 6. CRESO
_____ 7. lead-lined walls
_____ 8. 6 feet away
_____ 9. minimum scatter
_____ 10. barrier

Column B

a. right angles to the x-ray beam
b. 5000 mrem
c. not always necessary
d. 50 rem/year
e. radiation shielding
f. radiation survey
g. personal radiation exposure
h. filtration
i. 500 mrem
j. proper operator position
k. lead apron
l. behind the patient
m. pocket dosimeter

IV. COMPLETE THESE STATEMENTS

1. Three factors used in calculating the type of barrier needed in a dental office are _____, _____, and _____.

2. The two methods that can alert dental personnel to the amount of occupational exposure they are receiving are through a _____ and by wearing a _____.

3. The _____ is the calculated maximum accumulated lifetime dose of radiation that a dental professional can receive.

4. The MPD for occupational exposure to ionizing radiation will be _____.

5. If a pregnant operator follows proper procedure, there is _____ to the fetus.

6. _____ construction, if of proper thickness, is sufficient for proper radiation shielding.

7. A film badge reading of 400 mR for a 4-week period _____.

8. If one is positioned 6 feet from the head of the x-ray machine during an exposure, then _____.

9. Under no circumstance should the dental professional _____.

10. Operators should not wear their film badges _____ their offices.

V. MULTIPLE CHOICE

Select the best answer.

1. At present the recommended MPD for nonoccupationally exposed individuals is
   a. 500 mrem/year
   b. 5 mrem/year
   c. 5 rem/year
   d. 5000 mrem/year
   e. 0.5 mrem/year

2. The occupational radiation dose will be kept to zero if
   a. careful technique is employed
   b. the office is well designed
   c. the office is well monitored
   d. the office is well equipped
   e. All of the above are correct.

3. The MPD is best defined as
   a. the maximum dose of radiation a patient should receive from dental exposures
   b. the permissible amount of radiation that causes cancer in human populations
   c. the maximum dose of ionizing radiation that is not expected to cause injury
   d. the amount of radiation that kills 50% of a population in 30 days
   e. none of the above

4. By having the operator stand 6 feet rather than 3 feet from a radiation source, the resultant exposure is decreased by a factor of
   a. 2
   b. 4
   c. 6
   d. 8
   e. 10

5. The International Commission on Radiological Protection (ICRP) has recommended that the yearly MPD for operators not exceed
   a. 5 mrem
   b. 500 mrem
   c. 50 mrem
   d. 5000 mrem
   e. 5.5 mrem

6. Workload determination for dental x-ray machine room barriers requires knowledge of
   a. milliamperage
   b. exposure time per film
   c. number of exposures per week
   d. adjacent room location
   e. experience of operator
      (1) a, d, e
      (2) a, b, c
      (3) a, b, c, d
      (4) c, d, e
      (5) a, c, d, e

7. What can be used to check the reliability of the x-ray machine and protective barriers?
   a. film badge
   b. ionizing chamber
   c. pocket dosimeter
   d. coin test
   e. a, b, and c only

8. Which of the following is true regarding film badges?
   a. They should be worn when dental personnel have radiographs as a patient.
   b. Film badges can be shared by employees.
   c. Film badges can be worn outside the office.
   d. Film badges should be worn so they are not blocked by pens or jewelry.
   e. None of the above is correct.

9. Which of the following, if sufficient, could provide adequate shielding?
   a. lead-lined walls
   b. dry wall construction
   c. cinder block walls
   d. concrete walls
   e. All of the above could be adequate.

10. What is the main source of radiation exposure to the operator?
    a. primary radiation
    b. scatter radiation
    c. background radiation
    d. tertiary radiation
    e. none of the above

VI. TRUE/FALSE

Select whether each statement is true (**T**) or false (**F**). Circle the correct answer.

1. Operators of dental x-ray machines should be 4 feet away from the source of radiation. **T/F**
2. Lead-lined walls in a dental operatory are not mandatory. **T/F**
3. Film badges are always required in a dental office. **T/F**
4. The MPD for occupationally exposed individuals in the dental office per week is 100 mrem. **T/F**
5. Selection criteria are guidelines established to mandate barrier protection in the operatory. **T/F**

VII. ORDERING QUESTIONS

Place the numbers 1, 2, 3, 4, and 5 in the spaces provided below to indicate the proper ordering sequence for the following questions.

1. Put the following radiation protection measures for the dental radiographer to follow in the order that they should occur (from the first to the last):

   _____ The operator should not hold the receptor in the patient's mouth.

   _____ The operator should stand 6 feet away from the source of radiation.

   _____ The operator should not stand in back of the tube head or behind the patient.

   _____ The operator should be behind an acceptable barrier.

   _____ The operator should be sure that fellow workers are not in the path of x-radiation when pressing the exposure button.

2. Put the recommended MPDs for occupationally involved individuals and for the general public in order (from the least to the most):

   _____ National Council on Radiation Protection and Measurements (NCRP) recommendation for occupational exposure is 50 mSv (5000 mrem) per year.

   _____ ICRP recommendation for the general public is 1 mSv (100 mrem) per year.

   _____ ICRP recommendation for occupational exposure is 20 mSv (2000 mrem) per year.

   _____ NCRP recommendation for the general public is 5mSv (500 mrem) per year.

   _____ The CUMEfd (lifetime) for a 28-year-old's occupational exposure is 280 mSv (28,000 mrem).

3. Put the following factors for shielding or barrier requirements for dental radiography facilities in the order that they are evaluated (from first to last):

   _____ Use factor

   _____ Maximum kilovoltage

   _____ Workoad factor

   _____ Occupancy factor

   _____ Distance from the source of radiation (tube head)

Infection Control in Dental Radiography

After reading Chapter 8 of the textbook and completing this exercise, the student will be able to:
1. Define the key terms listed at the beginning of the chapter.
2. State the primary purpose of infection control procedures, discuss the significance of cross-contamination in the office setting, and summarize the significance of taking an accurate medical history of your patient.
3. Define the meaning of a *pathogen,* and explain its relevance to an infection control protocol in the dental office.
4. Describe what the term *personal protective equipment (PPE)* means in reference to dental office infection control programs, as well as what the advised PPE requirements are for dental radiography.
5. Discuss the barriers used for sterilization, disinfection, digital radiography, film packets, processing solutions, and panoramic radiography in the dental office. In addition, perform the following procedures and discuss infection control protocol for each:
   - Chairside Exposure Procedures
   - Processing Procedures (Conventional Radiography)
   - Procedure for Daylight Loaders
6. Decide when antibiotic prophylaxis is required for dental radiographic procedures and what vaccinations are required for dental personnel.

I. DEFINITIONS

Define/explain the following terms.

1. AIDS _____

_____

2. Barrier envelope _____

_____

3. CDC _____

_____

4. Cold sterilization _____

_____

5. Contamination _____

_____

6. Critical instruments _____

_____

7. Cross-contamination _____

_____

8. Disinfection _____

_____

9. Immunization _____

_____

10. Infection control barriers _____

_____

11. OSHA _____

_____

12. Parental exposure _____

_____

13. Pathogen _____

_____

14. PPE _____

_____

15. Universal precautions _____

_____

II. COMPREHENSION EXERCISE

1. In dental radiography what are the main vectors for cross-contamination?

2. What is the significance of taking a comprehensive medical history on a patient before dental treatment?

3. What are the required barriers that dental personnel must wear (PPE) while performing radiographic procedures?

4. What is the most appropriate barrier used for equipment in the operatory when performing radiography?

5. Why is saliva considered to be a possible transmission route for human immunodeficiency virus (HIV)?

6. What is the difference between sterilization and disinfection? How is each used in dental radiography?

7. For which diseases should dental personnel receive immunizations?

8. Describe the use of the processing solutions used in the darkroom in terms of the disinfection and sterilization of the film.

9. What are the infection control requirements concerning digital radiography in the dental office?

10. What are the cross-contamination hazards with the use of a daylight loader?

11. List the infection control procedures that operators should follow before, during, and after taking dental radiographs.

12. What is the general consensus regarding antibiotic prophylaxis and dental radiographic procedures?

13. Describe three ways to handle contaminated film packets to avoid contaminating the film.

14. What is a barrier film packet? Describe its use.

15. What type of infection control procedures is necessary when using an automatic processor with a daylight loader? Without a daylight loader?

55

16. What is "cold sterilization?" Is it appropriate for use in dental radiography?

17. What is the problem in using disinfecting solutions instead of barriers with the dental x-ray machine?

18. Discuss the advantages of using gloves, mask, and eyewear when performing dental radiographic procedures.

19. What are the infection control procedures needed when taking a panoramic radiograph?

20. Explain the following statement and its clinical significance: "All pathogens are microorganisms, but not all micro-organisms are pathogens."

III. MATCHING

Match the items in *Column A* with the appropriate items in *Column B*.

Column A

_____ 1. AIDS
_____ 2. immunization
_____ 3. pathogen
_____ 4. barriers
_____ 5. disinfecting solution
_____ 6. sterilization
_____ 7. cold sterilization
_____ 8. antiseptic agent
_____ 9. barrier envelope
_____ 10. saliva
_____ 11. previous endocarditis
_____ 12. semicritical instrument
_____ 13. critical instrument
_____ 14. occupational exposure
_____ 15. film packet

Column B

a. film
b. main vector
c. antibiotic prophylaxis
d. no vaccine
e. hepatitis B
f. contaminant
g. protects film
h. patient's chart
i. soap
j. periodontal probe
k. gloves, mask, eyewear, gowns
l. steam autoclave
m. iodophor
n. film-holding device
o. not recommended
p. causes disease

IV. COMPLETE THESE STATEMENTS

1. Even before the advent of AIDS, _____

   and _____ had always been a risk for dental professionals.

2. _____ is the most common and easily recognized transmission route of HIV, HBV, and HCV.

3. AIDS and HIV are abbreviations for _____

   and _____.

4. When taking intraoral radiographs, _____,

   _____, _____,

   and _____ should be worn at all times.

5. All dental professionals should be immunized for

   _____.

6. The most common methods of sterilization used in the

   dental office are _____

   and the use of the _____.

7. Infection control procedures require that every patient

   be treated _____.

8. Three vehicles for the transmission of pathogens on

   intraoral film holders are _____,

   _____, and

   _____.

9. Other than the operator's hands, the _____ is considered to be the main source of cross-contamination in dental radiography.

10. Anything that the operator touches after removing the exposed film packet from the patient's mouth must be

    considered _____.

11. All working surfaces and the dental x-ray unit should be _____ before radio-graphs are taken.

12. Digital sensors should be covered with _____ before use.

13. _____ can be contaminated by blood and therefore poses a potential for transmission of infectious organisms.

14. Film packets are considered _____ after they are removed from the patient's mouth.

15. The developing and fixing solutions used in the darkroom have not been shown to act as _____ agents.

V. MULTIPLE CHOICE

Select the best answer.

1. Which of the following infection control procedures is used in dental radiography?
   a. sterilization
   b. disinfection
   c. antiseptic agents
   d. instant hand sanitizer
   e. all of the above

2. If the barrier envelope is not used
   a. operators could open the packet without gloves
   b. operators should remove the films while wearing the same gloves used for exposure
   c. operators should take care not to touch the films as they are dropped onto a clean surface
   d. operators could touch anything on the way to the darkroom with the previously contaminated gloves
   e. none of the above

3. Daylight loaders are not recommended for infection control because of the
   a. strength of the processing solutions
   b. time delay
   c. possibility of cross-contamination within the confined area of the loader
   d. light leaks
   e. none of the above

4. Infection control procedures should be followed for
   a. patients known to have AIDS
   b. patients who are HIV positive
   c. patients with an alternative lifestyle
   d. all patients
   e. noncompliant patients

5. Any contaminated film that is processed
   a. emerges from the processor sterilized
   b. emerges from the processor disinfected
   c. emerges from the processor decontaminated
   d. emerges from the processor still contaminated
   e. none of the above

6. With the use of a barrier envelope
   a. no other precautions are necessary
   b. gloves are not necessary after the film has been removed from the packs
   c. processing is less difficult
   d. processing is more difficult
   e. an increased exposure time is needed

7. Developer and fixer solutions
   a. do not act as sterilizing agents
   b. are antiseptic
   c. act as sterilizing agents
   d. destroy all viruses
   e. none of the above

8. Autoclaving a contaminated exposed film packet
   a. is not recommended because it takes too long
   b. does not sterilize the packet
   c. destroys the image
   d. refines the image
   e. none of the above

9. Every patient should have a current medical history that
   a. is obtained through a questionnaire
   b. is obtained through direct questioning
   c. alerts the dental team to the presence or history of infectious disease
   d. All of the above are valid statements.
   e. None of the above are valid statements.

10. Immersing the contaminated exposed film packet in a disinfecting solution
    a. destroys the image
    b. is recommended
    c. takes too long
    d. none of the above
    e. all of the above

11. Using disinfecting solutions directly sprayed on the digital sensor and the keyboard is not recommended because
    a. of the cost involved
    b. of the time involved
    c. it is not effective
    d. the solution may affect the electrical connections
    e. none of the above

12. Microorganisms can remain viable on radiographic equipment for at least
    a. 72 hours
    b. 48 hours
    c. 10 hours
    d. 24 hours
    e. none of the above

13. When taking bitewings on a patient with a negative medical history
    a. gloves and eyewear should be used
    b. just gloves are necessary
    c. gloves, eyeglasses, protective clothing, and masks should be worn
    d. eyeglasses are not necessary
    e. none of the above

14. When taking a full-mouth series of radiographs
    a. the exposure switch should be covered with plastic
    b. the PID need not be covered if gloves are worn
    c. a film dispenser should not be used
    d. unexposed film should be kept in the room
    e. none of the above

15. The infection control procedure for daylight loaders includes
    a. preparing the interior of the daylight loader before processing
    b. placing clean hands through the sleeve baffles
    c. opening packets with clean gloves
    d. All of the above are true statements.
    e. None of the above are true statements.

VI. TRUE/FALSE

Select whether each statement is true (**T**) or false (**F**). Circle the correct answer.

1. An antiseptic is a substance that inhibits the growth of bacteria. **T/F**
2. Sterilization is the process of destroying disease-causing microorganisms by physical or chemical means. **T/F**
3. Every patient should not be treated in the same manner such as with universal precautions. **T/F**
4. The processing procedure for films with and without barrier envelopes is exactly the same. **T/F**
5. In panoramic radiography more areas are contaminated by the patient's saliva. **T/F**

VII. ORDERING QUESTIONS

Place the numbers 1, 2, 3, 4, and 5 in the spaces provided below to indicate the proper ordering sequence for the following questions.

1. Put the following chairside infection control procedures in the order that they are advised to occur (from the first to the last):

    _____ Wash hands thoroughly.

    _____ Take the prescribed exposures, taking care to touch only the covered surfaces.

    _____ Cover all appropriate surfaces with a plastic barrier.

    _____ Set out all supplies in advance.

    _____ Seat the patient and cover him or her with a cleaned and disinfected lead apron and thyroid collar.

2. Put the following infection control automatic processing procedures in the order that they are advised to occur (from the first to the last):

    _____ Remove the barrier envelopes from the exposed films.

    _____ Place the films in the automatic processor.

    _____ Expose all films.

    _____ Remove the gloves.

    _____ Open the film packets and dispose of the plastic wrapper, black paper wrapper, and lead foil backing.

3. Put the following digital radiography infection control procedures in the order that they are advised to occur (from the first to the last):

    _____ Cover all surfaces with plastic barriers, including the tube head, control panel, on/off switch, and keyboard.

    _____ Take the prescribed exposures.

    _____ Wipe the digital sensor and wire with a disinfectant.

    _____ Cover the sensor with an appropriate barrier protective sheath.

    _____ Throw away all contaminated barriers and wipe the sensor before storing it.

9 Intraoral Radiographic Technique: The Paralleling Method

EDUCATIONAL OBJECTIVES

After reading Chapter 9 of the textbook and completing this exercise, the student will be able to:

1. Define the key terms listed at the beginning of the chapter.
2. Discuss the following related to the radiographic survey:
   - Know the importance of radiographs in treatment planning and diagnosis.
   - Explain what factors are involved in "prescribing" dental radiographs.
   - State the components of a general full-mouth survey (FMS), a pediatric FMS, and an edentulous FMS.
   - Describe what should be seen on periapical and bitewing projections and what the indications for use are for both projections.
   - Know the 8 criteria for acceptable intraoral radiographs.
3. List the principles, advantages, and disadvantages of the paralleling technique.
4. Recite the routine in preparing for and exposing dental radiographs, and explain the purpose of having a systematic sequence when exposing radiographic images.
5. Discuss the advantage of using a paralleling receptor-holding device (i.e., extension cone paralleling [XCP] instrument) when exposing intraoral radiographs.
6. Discuss the following related to the paralleling method:
   - List the six factors that must be considered in any periapical projection.
   - Know what factors are considered in determining the exposure time setting for dental radiographic exposures.
   - Be able to apply the principles of the paralleling intraoral radiographic technique to exposing all periapical and bitewing radiographs indicated for their dental patients.
7. Know the causes, appearances, and remedies for the discussed exposure errors, as well as list the three most common bitewing errors, including their causes, appearance, and remedies.

I. DEFINITIONS

Define/explain the following terms.

1. Bitewing radiograph _____

_____

2. Blurred image _____

_____

3. Collimator cutoff (cone cutting) _____

_____

4. Dimensional accuracy _____

_____

5. Double exposure _____

_____

6. Exposure time _____

_____

7. Film reversal _____

_____

8. Full-mouth survey (series) _____

_____

9. Horizontal angulation _____

_____

10. Localizing ring _____

_____

11. Overexposure _____

_____

12. Overlapping _____

_____

13. Paralleling method _____

_____

14. Patient movement _____

_____

15. Periapical radiograph _____

_____

16. Point of entry _____

_____

17. Sagittal plane orientation _____

_____

18. Underexposure _____

_____

19. Vertical angulation _____

_____

20. Vertical bitewing radiograph _____

_____

Chapter **9** Intraoral Radiographic Technique: The Paralleling Method

II. COMPREHENSION EXERCISE

1. Explain why it is necessary in a full-mouth series to take radiographs of edentulous areas.

2. What would be the indication for use of vertical bitewing projections?

3. Describe what an elongated radiograph looks like.

4. What is the importance of correct horizontal angulation?

5. List/explain two helpful hints for placement of the mandibular anterior projection.

6. What are the two main principles of the paralleling method?

7. What is the purpose of using a localizing ring?

8. Describe the receptor position for a maxillary molar projection.

9. How does the consequence of inadequate closure appear on a radiograph?

10. Describe what a foreshortened radiograph would look like.

11. Why does the operator remove nonfixed appliances from the patient's mouth when taking radiographs?

12. What can cause a blurred image?

13. Name three chairside technique errors that will result in a thin (light) image.

14. How does a cracked emulsion due to overbending the film packet appear on the radiograph?

15. List the criteria that determine whether a radiograph is considered diagnostic.

16. Why isn't there superimposition of the zygomatic arch on maxillary molars in the paralleling technique?

17. Can the paralleling method be used with an 8-inch target-receptor distance (FFD)? Explain.

18. What determines how many projections there will be in a pediatric full-mouth survey?

19. List/describe one way to avoid double-exposed projections.

20. What action would you take before using the bisecting-angle technique if parallel positioning of the receptor is difficult on a pediatric patient?

III. MATCHING

Match the items in *Column A* with the appropriate items in *Column B*.

Column A

_____ 1. proximal surface overlap
_____ 2. collimator cutoff
_____ 3. dense image
_____ 4. "herringbone" effect
_____ 5. thin image (light)
_____ 6. localizing ring
_____ 7. elongation
_____ 8. bitewing projection
_____ 9. residual pathology
_____ 10. loss of definition
_____ 11. bisecting-angle technique
_____ 12. 16-inch PID
_____ 13. inadequate vertical angulation
_____ 14. premolar projection
_____ 15. excessive vertical angulation

Column B

a. patient movement
b. overexposure
c. dimensional distortion
d. elongation
e. long cone technique
f. distal of the canine
g. beam-receptor alignment
h. image of an edentulous area
i. foreshortening
j. inadequate milliamperage
k. film reversal
l. unexposed image area
m. vertical angulation
n. patient tolerance
o. horizontal angulation
p. interproximal caries detection
q. identification dot

IV. COMPLETE THESE STATEMENTS

1. In using the paralleling method, the most appropriate FFD is _____.

2. An example of a film holder for intraoral periapical radiography is a _____ or _____.

3. _____ is determined by the area being radiographed, film speed, kilovoltage, milliamperage, and FFD.

4. Bitewing radiographs do not show the _____.

5. A black, crescent-shaped mark on a radiograph is an indication of _____.

6. The occlusal plane of the jaw being radiographed should be _____ to the floor.

7. The location on the patient's face that corresponds to the center of the film is called the _____.

8. Failure to align the x-ray beam with the film packet will result in _____.

9. If the film packet is curved to accommodate the shape of the palate, it should be curved _____ the source of radiation.

10. Another name for the paralleling method is _____.

11. The sagittal plane of the patient's face always should be _____.

12. The film packet should be placed _____ to both the vertical and horizontal axis of the tooth being radiographed.

13. When taking a full-mouth series, partial dentures always should be _____ to avoid superimposition.

14. Increasing the FFD without changing the milliamperage will result in a _____.

15. The most common error in the paralleling technique is in _____.

V. MULTIPLE CHOICE

Select the best answer.

1. A reason for using the paralleling method instead of the bisecting method is
   a. less thyroid dose to the patient
   b. less dimensional distortion
   c. less exit dose
   d. no superimposition of the zygomatic arch
   e. all of the above

2. Bitewing radiographs are used to detect
   a. periodontal bone loss
   b. interproximal caries
   c. recurrent caries
   d. the ill fit of metallic restorations
   e. all of the above

3. In taking the radiograph, you did not center the beam on the receptor in the patient's mouth. The resulting film will show
   a. fogging
   b. overlapping
   c. elongation
   d. collimator cutoff
   e. foreshortening

4. A set of radiographs all show thin images. One possible error that could have caused this is
   a. the developing solution is too hot
   b. excessive milliampere seconds
   c. excessive kilovoltage peak
   d. excessive FFD
   e. excessive developing time

5. If a film packet is placed in the patient's mouth with the wrong side facing the x-ray beam, the resulting film will
   a. be blank
   b. have a thin image
   c. be overexposed
   d. show no effect
   e. have a thin image with a geometric pattern on it

6. The failure to remove partial dentures while taking radiographs may cause
   a. collimator cutoff
   b. a blurred image
   c. superimposition of the metallic object on the film
   d. overlapped images
   e. double exposure

7. A "long cone" (16-inch FFD) is used in the paralleling technique to
   a. reduce secondary radiation
   b. avoid magnification of the image
   c. avoid distortion of the image
   d. avoid superimposition of the zygomatic arch
   e. facilitate correct vertical angulation

8. Using a localizing ring with a receptor holder helps in preventing
   a. collimator cutoff
   b. elongation
   c. foreshortening
   d. overlapping
   e. overexposure

9. The projection most likely to excite the gag reflex is the
   a. mandibular molar projection
   b. maxillary molar projection
   c. molar bitewing projection
   d. premolar bitewing projection
   e. maxillary canine projection

10. The best way to prevent patient movement during intraoral radiography is
    a. fast film
    b. short PIDs
    c. good operator technique
    d. high kilovoltage
    e. high milliamperage

11. In using a receptor-holding device with a localizing ring, it is not necessary that
    a. the occlusal plane be parallel to the floor
    b. the sagittal plane be perpendicular to the floor
    c. the backrest be elevated
    d. the headrest be under the occiput
    e. all of the above

12. A full-mouth survey
    a. always has periapical and bitewing projections
    b. has a minimum of 20 images
    c. varies in need and number of images according to selection criteria and mouth size
    d. can be replaced in all cases by a panoramic projection
    e. none of the above

13. Another correct way to refer to the paralleling method is
    a. short cone technique
    b. right-angle technique
    c. periapical method
    d. bitewing method
    e. none of the above

14. In order to avoid creating an artifact on the apex of the tooth when placing the film in the film holder, which of the following statements is accurate?
    a. "The dot" should be away from "the slot."
    b. "The dot" should be on the opposite the side of "the slot."
    c. It doesn't matter where "the dot" is placed.
    d. "The dot" should be in "the slot."
    e. Placement of "the dot" depends on the projection being taken.

15. Placement of the premolar projection should include
    a. the first and second premolars
    b. most of the first molar
    c. the distal of the canine
    d. only the first and second premolars
    e. a, b, and c

VI. TRUE/FALSE

Select whether each statement is true (**T**) or false (**F**). Circle the correct answer.

1. A bitewing film shows the entire tooth from the occlusal surface or incisal edge to the apex of the tooth. **T/F**
2. The basic principle of the paralleling technique is that the tooth and film should be parallel to each other. **T/F**
3. The use of film holders is strongly discouraged in intraoral radiography. **T/F**
4. The most common exposure error in the paralleling technique is in receptor placement. **T/F**
5. Blurred images are the result of reversing the film in the patient's mouth. **T/F**

VII. ORDERING QUESTIONS

Place the numbers 1, 2, 3, 4, and 5 in the spaces provided below to indicate the proper ordering sequence for the following questions.

1. Put the following list of criteria for acceptable intraoral radiographs in the order they are listed (from first to last):

   _____ All interproximal surfaces should be seen without overlapping.

   _____ The radiograph should not be bent.

   _____ The radiograph should show proper definition and detail.

   _____ The structures of the teeth on the radiograph should not be elongated or foreshortened.

   _____ The periapical radiograph should show the entire tooth plus 2-3 mm of surrounding bone.

2. Put the following projections in the exposure order that is recommended (from first to last):

_____ Maxillary molar projection

_____ Premolar bitewing projection

_____ Mandibular incisors projection

_____ Maxillary canine projection

_____ Mandibular premolar projection

3. Put the following steps in the radiographic exposure routine in the order that is recommended (from first to last):

_____ The patient is seated.

_____ The patient is draped with a lead apron and thyroid collar.

_____ The patient is asked to remove any metallic objects that will interfere with the radiographic procedure.

_____ The proper infection control procedures should be followed.

_____ The prescribed radiographs are exposed.

Accessory Radiographic Techniques: Bisecting Technique and Occlusal Projections

10

EDUCATIONAL OBJECTIVES

After reading Chapter 10 of the textbook and completing this exercise, the student will be able to:

1. Define the key terms listed at the beginning of the chapter.
2. Discuss the following related to the bisecting technique:
   - Know the basic principles of the bisecting technique.
   - State the indication for use of the bisecting technique as an accessory intraoral radiographic technique.
   - List and explain the advantages and disadvantages of the bisecting technique.
   - Describe the three methods of utilizing the bisecting technique.
3. List and describe the two most common errors produced with the use of incorrect vertical angulation in the bisecting technique, as well as the remedies for each.
4. Discuss the following related to occlusal film projections:
   - State the purpose and the indications for use of the occlusal exposure technique in dental intraoral radiography.
   - State the two types of occlusal projections and what each is generally used for in dental radiography.
   - List the steps involved in preparation and exposure of occlusal projections on the dental patient.
   - State the recommended vertical angulation for the maxillary and mandibular right-angle and topographic occlusal projections.

I. DEFINITIONS

Define/explain the following terms.

1. Anatomical constraints _____

_____

2. Bisecting-angle technique _____

_____

3. Buccolingual dimension _____

_____

4. Dimensional distortion _____

_____

5. Elongated image _____

_____

6. Foreshortened image _____

_____

7. Imaginary bisecting line _____

_____

8. Headrest position _____

_____

9. Horizontal angulation _____

_____

10. Negative angulation _____

_____

11. Occlusal receptor _____

_____

12. Occlusal plane orientation _____

_____

13. Occlusal projection _____

_____

14. Overlapped image _____

_____

15. Positive angulation _____

_____

16. Receptor plane _____

_____

17. Right-angle occlusal projection _____

_____

18. Sagittal plane orientation _____

_____

19. Topographic occlusal projection _____

_____

II. COMPREHENSION EXERCISE

1. Describe the advantages of the bisecting technique as compared to the paralleling technique.

2. What generally is the indication for use of an occlusal projection? What are the specific indications for topographic versus right-angle projections?

3. Describe the disadvantages of the bisecting technique when compared to the paralleling technique.

4. Describe the method used with the bisecting-angle technique.

5. Explain the difference between horizontal angulation and vertical angulation.

6. In the bisecting technique, what dictates the point of entry?

7. Why is the thyroid dose higher in the bisecting technique than in the paralleling technique?

8. In intraoral radiography, what is the correct sagittal plane orientation for the patient's head?

9. Why does the bisecting technique call for an 8-inch target-receptor distance (FFD)?

10. In the bisecting technique, what determines the variations in vertical angulation from one projection to another?

11. Explain why it is necessary to use occlusal projections when localizing impacted teeth.

12. In an edentulous survey, what is the main reason for using topographic occlusal projections? Name two alternatives.

13. Why is the use of shorter exposure times with the bisecting technique not valid as an advantage at this point in time?

14. In the bisecting technique, why is occlusal plane orientation so critical?

15. Explain why the topographic occlusal projection is said to be a modification of the bisecting technique.

III. MATCHING

Match the items in *Column A* with the appropriate items in *Column B*.

Column A

_____ 1. elongation
_____ 2. buccolingual localization
_____ 3. 8-inch FFD
_____ 4. poor sagittal plane orientation
_____ 5. foreshortening
_____ 6. higher thyroid dose
_____ 7. occlusal plane
_____ 8. overlapped image
_____ 9. greater exit dose
_____ 10. short buccal image structure
_____ 11. dimensional accuracy
_____ 12. large pathologic areas
_____ 13. positive angulation
_____ 14. negative angulation
_____ 15. #4 size receptor

Column B

a. bisecting technique
b. parallel to the floor
c. dimensional distortion
d. topographic occlusal
e. poor horizontal angulation
f. image magnification
g. insufficient vertical angulation
h. occlusal receptor size
i. too much vertical angulation
j. periapical receptor size
k. right-angle occlusal projection
l. mandibular arch
m. fogged image
n. elongation
o. maxillary arch
p. 8-inch target = FFD
q. paralleling technique

IV. COMPLETE THESE STATEMENTS

1. The projection of choice to completely visualize a palatal lesion would be _____.

2. The dose to the thyroid gland is _____ in the bisecting technique when compared to the paralleling technique because of _____.

3. The correct chair position for the bisecting technique requires that the sagittal plane of the patient's face is _____ to the floor.

4. The anatomic landmark for the point of entry for the mandibular bicuspid periapical film is the _____.

5. Periodontal bone height may be exaggerated in the bisecting technique because of _____.

6. In the bisecting technique, an overly dense image may be caused by _____ or _____.

7. Foreshortening can be caused by excessive vertical angulation or poor _____ orientation.

8. Two projections other than periapical projections that can be used in an edentulous survey of the mandible are _____ and _____.

9. Usually the FFD used in the paralleling technique is _____ than in the bisecting technique.

10. The major disadvantage of the bisecting technique is that the image projected on the receptor is _____.

11. The vertical angulation for the maxillary incisors in the bisecting technique would be about _____ degrees.

12. In the bisecting technique, the receptor should be held in the patient's mouth with a _____.

13. Horizontal angulation is established so that the _____ is perpendicular to the receptor in the _____ plane.

14. Occlusal film has the _____ speed (sensitivity) as periapical film size #2.

15. The angulation of the _____ may vary from 45 to 75 degrees, depending on the anatomic area.

V. MULTIPLE CHOICE

Select the best answer.

1. You have decided to change the position-indicating device (PID) in your office, replacing the 16-inch cylinder with an 8-inch cylinder. The milliamperage will remain the same, as will the kilovolt peak value. The old exposure time for mandibular molars was 36 impulses; the new exposure time to obtain images of equal density will be
   a. 12 impulses
   b. 24 impulses
   c. 18 impulses
   d. 9 impulses
   e. 48 impulses

2. The posterior topographic view of the maxilla can be considered a topographic view of the
   a. zygoma
   b. maxillary sinus
   c. zygomatic process
   d. maxillary tuberosity
   e. none of the above

3. In taking a periapical radiograph using the bisecting technique, the x-ray beam was not centered on the receptor. The resulting image shows
   a. fogging
   b. overlapping
   c. collimator cutoff
   d. foreshortening
   e. elongation

4. In taking a periapical radiograph of the maxillary incisor area by the bisecting technique, using a vertical angulation of +15 degrees will result in an image that
   a. has collimator cutoff
   b. is foreshortened
   c. is elongated
   d. is overlapped
   e. is correct

5. When using the bisecting-angle technique for a maxillary premolar projection, the point of entry is
   a. the base of the lateral nasal groove
   b. just below the midpoint of the nares
   c. the most anterior part of the cheekbone
   d. the zygomatic arch
   e. none of the above

6. The best way to visualize a salivary stone in the floor of the mouth is by using a
   a. panoramic projection
   b. maxillary occlusal projection
   c. mandibular central incisor projection
   d. mandibular right-angle occlusal projection
   e. mandibular topographic occlusal projection

7. Occlusal film is classified as size
   a. #2
   b. #0
   c. #4
   d. #3
   e. #1

8. For the maxillary molar periapical projection, the center of the receptor should be aligned with
   a. the junction between the first and second molars
   b. the middle of the first molar
   c. the junction between the second and third molars
   d. the middle of the second molar
   e. none of the above

9. In the bisecting technique, if the central ray is not perpendicular to the receptor in the horizontal plane, the resulting image will be
   a. foreshortened
   b. overlapped
   c. "cone cut"
   d. elongated
   e. blurred

10. Using the bisecting technique in taking a periapical radiograph of tooth #32, using a vertical angulation of −30 degrees will result in an image that is
    a. foreshortened
    b. overlapped
    c. elongated
    d. "cone cut"
    e. reversed

11. What would be the projection of choice to visualize a large lesion in the midline of the palate?
    a. panoramic
    b. maxillary right-angle occlusal
    c. maxillary topographic occlusal
    d. maxillary molar periapical
    e. maxillary incisor periapical

12. When using the bisecting technique, the point of entry for the mandibular molar projection is the
    a. roots of the molars
    b. root of the first molar
    c. cemento-enamel junction of the molars
    d. crowns of the molars
    e. bifurcation of the second molar

13. The film speed of occlusal film is
    a. slower than periapical film
    b. the same as periapical film
    c. faster than bitewing film
    d. the same as panoramic film
    e. faster than periapical film

14. The best projection to decide whether an impacted maxillary canine is located bucally or lingually is the
    a. maxillary topographic occlusal
    b. panoramic
    c. canine periapical using the paralleling method
    d. canine periapical using the bisecting method
    e. maxillary right-angle occlusal

15. The bisecting-angle technique may be an advantageous technique to use with
    a. small children
    b. people with low palatal vaults
    c. patients with small mouths
    d. patients with anatomic constraints prohibiting the use of paralleling devices
    e. all of the above

VI. TRUE/FALSE

Select whether each statement is true (**T**) or false (**F**). Circle the correct answer.

1. In the bisecting technique, the receptor is placed parallel to the occlusal surfaces of the teeth being radiographed. **T/F**
2. The major disadvantage of the bisecting technique is dimensional distortion. **T/F**
3. In the bisecting technique, the central ray is directed perpendicular to an imaginary bisecting line between the tooth and receptor. **T/F**
4. Foreshortening is a result of overbending of the film packet in the bisecting technique. **T/F**
5. Occlusal radiographs are seldom taken to view salivary stones in the submandibular gland. **T/F**

Chapter **10** **Accessory Radiographic Techniques: Bisecting Technique and Occlusal Projections**

VII. ORDERING QUESTIONS

Place the numbers 1, 2, 3, 4, and 5 in the spaces provided below to indicate the proper ordering sequence for the following questions.

1. Put the following principles of the bisecting technique in their acceptable order (from first to last):

    _____ The receptor is placed as close to the tooth as possible.

    _____ An 8-inch FFD is used.

    _____ The vertical angle is set so that the central ray is perpendicular to an imaginary bisector.

    _____ The object-receptor distance is minimal.

    _____ No compensation for image enlargement is necessary.

2. Put the following steps used in the third method of utilizing the bisecting technique in the order that is recommended by the text (from first to last):

    _____ Check the vertical angle setting on the yolk of the x-ray unit.

    _____ Divide the noted vertical angle in half.

    _____ Place the receptor in a simple receptor-holding device and as close to the teeth being radiographed as possible.

    _____ Set the central ray (PID) so that it is perpendicular to the receptor.

    _____ Reset the vertical angulation at that halfway setting and expose the projection.

3. Put the following exposure factors for the bisecting technique in the recommended order (from first to last):

    _____ Point of entry

    _____ Receptor position

    _____ Chair position

    _____ Horizontal angulation

    _____ Vertical angulation

11 Film Processing Techniques

I. DEFINITIONS

Define/explain the following terms.

1. Archival life _____

_____

2. Automatic processing _____

_____

3. Clear film _____

_____

4. Coin test _____

_____

5. Darkroom _____

_____

6. Daylight loader _____

_____

7. Developer cutoff _____

_____

8. Film fog _____

_____

9. Film hangers _____

_____

10. Latent image _____

_____

11. Manual processing _____

_____

12. Rapid processing _____

_____

13. Reference film _____

_____

14. Replenisher solutions _____

_____

15. Safelight _____

_____

16. Sight developing _____

_____

17. Silver retrieval _____

_____

18. Thermostatic valve _____

_____

19. Time-temperature processing _____

_____

20. Visible image _____

_____

II. COMPREHENSION EXERCISE

1. List, describe, and state the purpose of each step involved in the manual processing of dental x-ray film.

2. What is the primary precaution that should be taken when processing extraoral radiographs? Why?

3. How do you test for safelight reliability?

4. Why is the time-temperature technique the best method for processing radiographs?

5. List and explain the three types of wastes that can be generated as a result of dental radiography.

6. Is sight developing an acceptable technique? Why or why not?

7. Why is it not acceptable to underdevelop a film to compensate for overexposure of the same film?

8. What is the major advantage of automatic processing? Explain.

9. List the chemicals that make up the developer and fixer solutions and identify the function of each.

10. What are the clinical indications for rapid processing? What are the disadvantages?

11. List two ways to check the strength of the processing solutions as a component of the quality assurance program and explain each method.

12. When must safelight conditions be maintained in the darkroom?

13. What are the responsibilities of the dental support team in the darkroom?

14. Define reticulation and describe the cause and remedy related to this processing error.

15. Distinguish between the appearance of collimator cutoff (cone cutting) and developer cutoff on the finished radiograph.

16. Can one distinguish between an overexposed film and an overdeveloped film? How?

17. What can cause a clear film?

18. Discuss the importance of a quality assurance program in the darkroom.

19. When should processing solutions be changed?

20. What causes white lines on a finished radiograph? Black lines?

21. What will happen if film is left in the fixer solution over a weekend?

22. What should you do if succeeding panoramic films appear increasingly light?

23. Why is it important to maintain the levels of the processing solutions? How often should the levels be checked? What should be done to maintain the adequate levels?

24. If the temperature of the developing solution is cold, how will the time needed for adequate development be affected? What if the temperature of the developing solution is hot? Explain your answers.

25. Name the five different light sources in a well-designed darkroom and provide the purpose for each.

III. MATCHING

Match the items in *Column A* with the appropriate items in *Column B*.

Column A

_____ 1. coin test
_____ 2. lost films in tank
_____ 3. underdeveloped film
_____ 4. static marks
_____ 5. excessive fixing
_____ 6. overdeveloped film
_____ 7. energized silver bromide
_____ 8. radiolucent bands on film
_____ 9. sodium carbonate
_____ 10. thermometer
_____ 11. air bubbles
_____ 12. unaffected silver bromide
_____ 13. energized silver
_____ 14. overlapped films
_____ 15. change solutions

Column B

a. latent image
b. agitate film hangers
c. dense image
d. 2 to 3 weeks
e. softens gelatin
f. films fed too quickly
g. hardens gelatin crystals
h. clear films
i. thin image
j. safelight check
k. dirty rollers
l. "wet elbow"
m. fixer precipitated
n. forcefully open packet
o. developer
p. reticulation
q. kept in the developer

IV. COMPLETE THESE STATEMENTS

1. The temperature of the processing chemicals is maintained by _____.

2. If the developer solution contaminates the fixer solution, the operator should _____.

3. Two types of light used in the darkroom are _____ and _____.

4. Two advantages of automatic processors are _____ and _____.

5. A latent image is invisible until the film is _____.

6. The easiest way to check a darkroom for light leaks is to _____.

7. At minimum, developer and fixer levels should be checked _____.

8. A manually processed radiograph should be washed for _____ just before drying.

9. The thermometer in a darkroom is always kept in the _____ solution.

10. The levels of the processing chemicals should be maintained by adding _____.

11. Expended fixer solution should be disposed of by _____.

12. To determine whether a safelight is "safe," one should _____.

13. X-ray processing solutions should be stored in a _____, _____ area.

14. For complete fixation, the films should be left in the solution for approximately _____ the developing time.

15. Panoramic films are processed in _____ as intraoral films.

V. MULTIPLE CHOICE

1. Each successive full-mouth survey appears lighter than the one before. Which of the following corrections should be made?
   a. Increase the mA setting.
   b. Increase the kV setting.
   c. Change the intensifying screens.
   d. Change the developer solution.
   e. Decrease the temperature of the developer solution.

2. A major difference between automatic and manual processing of radiographs is that automatic processing
   a. is more expensive
   b. provides better quality films
   c. requires special solutions at higher temperatures
   d. doesn't allow for processing errors
   e. allows for more latitude in exposure techniques

3. In developing radiographs, the fixer acts to
   a. prevent film fog and soften the emulsion
   b. remove exposed silver halide and soften the emulsion
   c. remove exposed silver halide and shrink and harden the emulsion
   d. remove unexposed and undeveloped silver halide from the film and harden the emulsion
   e. prevent reticulation and harden the emulsion

4. If the temperature of the processing solutions is slightly above normal, radiographs of desired density may be best obtained by
   a. increasing the fixing time
   b. decreasing the fixing time
   c. increasing the developing time
   d. decreasing the developing time
   e. increasing the exposure time

5. A latent image is
   a. found only on E-speed film
   b. caused only by scattered radiation
   c. prevented by the lead foil in the film packet
   d. invisible until the film is processed
   e. none of the above

6. An exposed radiograph should remain in the fixer in order to attain archival life
   a. for as long as it remains in the developer
   b. until the film clears
   c. for twice the developing time
   d. for a minimum of 1 hour
   e. for 5 minutes at 70°F

7. Which of the following causes dark spots during film development?
   a. film contamination with fixer before processing
   b. film contamination with developer before processing
   c. developing solution that is too warm
   d. overdevelopment of the exposed film
   e. none of the above

8. The effect of safelight illumination in the darkroom does not depend on which of the following?
   a. size of the darkroom
   b. type of film used
   c. wattage of the bulb
   d. type of filter used
   e. distance of the safelight from the work surface

9. A radiograph is clear after processing. This could result from any of the following *except*
   a. unexposed film
   b. excessive washing
   c. prolonged fixing
   d. exposure to white light
   e. the x-ray machine was not turned on

10. In treating an emergency patient, you remove the radiograph from the fixer bath after 3 minutes and wash it. It is diagnostic. After treatment the film is dried and put in the patient's chart.
    a. This is proper procedure.
    b. This is acceptable procedure.
    c. The film will turn yellowish-brown in a few weeks.
    d. The film should have been returned to the water bath overnight.
    e. None of the above is true.

11. The operator observes that a portion of the processed panoramic radiograph is completely black. What is the most likely cause?
    a. excessive exposure time
    b. exposure to white light
    c. exposure to a light leak
    d. temperature of the developer was too high
    e. patient movement occurred during exposure

12. In the time-temperature method of processing dental radiographs, the thermometer is
    a. not used
    b. kept in the fixer bath
    c. kept in the water bath
    d. kept in the developer bath
    e. not read for the first series processed

13. Which is the correct order for manually processing radiographs?
    a. rinse, develop, fix
    b. develop, fix, wash, dry
    c. develop, rinse, fix, wash, dry
    d. fix, rinse, develop, wash, dry
    e. None of the above is correct.

14. Even though proper exposure techniques were employed, radiographs emerging from an automatic processor exhibit chalky smudges. What is the most likely cause?
    a. improper safelighting
    b. use of outdated film
    c. premature contact with the developer solution
    d. premature contact with the fixer solution
    e. dirty processor rollers

15. Manufacturers recommend that radiographic developing solutions be covered to prevent
    a. evaporation of the solutions
    b. an increase in the strength of the solutions
    c. emission of an oxidizing agent
    d. dilution of the solutions
    e. both a and c are acceptable answers

16. The coin test of a safelight in the darkroom shows a clear outline of the coin. What does this mean?
    a. The developer is exhausted.
    b. The safelight is adequate.
    c. The fixer solution is weak.
    d. The safelight is faulty.
    e. There was inadequate fixation.

17. If films are fed into the automatic processor too rapidly, what can happen?
    a. Films will stick together.
    b. Films will be cracked.
    c. Static electricity will be generated.
    d. Radiographs will be lighter than normal.
    e. Radiographs will be darker than normal.

18. A step-wedge control device would be primarily used
    a. to test the safelight in the darkroom
    b. to evaluate the amount of radiation exposure
    c. to wedge steps of lead into the dental walls to act as a barrier to radiation
    d. for quality assurance of processing solutions
    e. to compare the dental films of one patient to another

19. Which of the following conditions will result in a radiograph that is too light?
    a. The darkroom door is left opened during developing.
    b. Processing solutions are too warm.
    c. The safelight is inadequate.
    d. The automatic processor has a daylight loader.
    e. The developing solution is too weak.

20. Which of the following does not cause film fog in developed radiographs?
    a. underexposure
    b. scatter radiation
    c. improper safelighting
    d. a light leak in the darkroom
    e. processing solutions that are too warm

21. After developing a complete radiographic series, the operator notices that the films on the bottom of the rack are of a different density than those at the top of the rack and concludes that
    a. the developing solution was contaminated
    b. the thermometer is faulty
    c. the fixer solution was reaching exhaustion
    d. the solutions were not stirred
    e. the developing solution was too cold

22. Your last patient before the weekend is a new patient on whom you take a full-mouth series of radiographs. If you process the films that evening,
    a. the films can be left in the water bath
    b. the films can be left in the fixer
    c. the films have to be processed immediately to preserve the latent image
    d. the films can be left in the developer
    e. the films must be processed completely and left to dry

23. One indication for "rapid processing" would be
    a. detection of caries
    b. periodontal bone evaluation
    c. confirming an endodontic measurement
    d. evaluating periapical changes
    e. none of the above

24. The action of the fixer on unenergized silver bromide crystals in the emulsion is to
    a. precipitate them as free silver
    b. fix them to the film base
    c. incorporate them into the hardened gelatin
    d. remove them from the film
    e. reuse them

85

25. Processing solutions should be changed, depending on usage, about
    a. every week
    b. every day
    c. every month
    d. every 2 to 3 weeks
    e. every 6 months

VI. TRUE/FALSE

Select whether each statement is true (**T**) or false (**F**). Circle the correct answer.

1. Automatic processing is never recommended over manual processing. **T/F**
2. When processing solutions are at a low level, water should be added. **T/F**
3. Expended fixing solutions should be poured down the drain. **T/F**
4. Sight development is a scientifically acceptable procedure of processing. **T/F**
5. The coin test is used to test the level of solutions in the processing tanks. **T/F**

VII. ORDERING QUESTIONS

Place the numbers 1, 2, 3, 4, and 5 in the spaces provided below to indicate the proper ordering sequence for the following questions.

1. Put the following steps in manually processing radiographic film in the order that they are recommended to occur (from first to last):

    _____ Stir the solutions.

    _____ Turn off the white light and turn on the safelight.

    _____ Open the film packets and put the films on the hangers.

    _____ The films are properly fixed, dried, and then mounted.

    _____ Immerse the film hanger in the developer, keeping it in the developer solution for the appropriate time.

2. Put the following steps in automatic processing radiographic film in the order that they are recommended to occur (from first to last) when the automatic processor does not have a daylight loader:

    _____ Retrieve the dried films and place them in a mount.

    _____ Make sure the processor is on and in the ready mode, not in the standby mode.

    _____ Go into the darkroom, lock the door, and turn off the lights, leaving only the safelight on.

    _____ Open the film packets.

    _____ Place them into the automatic processor slowly and not one behind the other.

3. Put the following steps in the processing of film from the latent image to the visible image in the order that they occur (from first to last):

    _____ The radiographic film is brought into the darkroom.

    _____ The fixer solution removes the unaffected crystals and leaves black, white, and gray areas.

    _____ The development process is complete and energized silver is precipitated as black areas.

    _____ The development process is started when the energized crystals are precipitated as free silver or black areas.

    _____ The latent image contains energized crystals that are shaded gray.

12 Panoramic Radiography

EDUCATIONAL OBJECTIVES

After reading Chapter 12 of the textbook and completing this exercise, the student will be able to:
1. Define the key terms listed at the beginning of the chapter.
2. Discuss the purpose of panoramic radiography.
3. Know the significance of the slit beam in panoramic radiography.
4. Explain the basics of panoramic radiography, including the importance of a focal trough or image layer.
5. Describe concepts related to pantomograms:
   - Describe how a panoramic image is produced.
   - List the positioning requirements for panoramic images.
   - Define *ghost image,* and explain its role in panoramic radiography.
6. List the advantages and disadvantages of panoramic imaging.
7. Discuss the main indications for use of a panoramic radiograph, and describe the interpretation of the images produced.
8. Know the cause, appearance, and remedy for technique errors in panoramic radiography.
9. Discuss the common contemporary artifacts that can be found on panoramic images.

I. DEFINITIONS

Define/explain the following terms.

1. Ala-tragus line _____

_____

2. Digital imaging _____

_____

3. Electrostatic artifact _____

_____

4. Focal trough _____

_____

5. Frankfort horizontal plane _____

_____

6. Ghost image _____

_____

7. Image layer _____

_____

8. Midsagittal plane _____

_____

9. Panoramic radiography _____

_____

10. "Panorex" _____

_____

11. Pantomograph _____

_____

12. Point of rotation _____

_____

13. Slit beam _____

_____

14. Tomographic cut _____

_____

15. Tomography _____

_____

II. COMPREHENSION EXERCISE

1. What are the advantages of a panoramic radiograph when compared to a full-mouth intraoral survey?

2. What are the disadvantages of a panoramic radiograph when compared to a full-mouth intraoral survey?

3. What does the term "panorama" mean? What is the term's significance in panoramic radiography?

4. Why is the patient's position so important in panoramic radiography?

5. How is patient movement avoided in panoramic radiography?

6. What are the two techniques available that produce panoramic images? Which technique is more widely used? Why?

7. What special precautions are necessary when processing panoramic films?

8. In panoramic radiography, what is a ghost image? How can it be avoided?

9. How can panoramic units be used to take tomograms of the temporomandibular joint (TMJ)?

10. What is the focal trough?

11. What is a "computer-driven tomographic unit?"

12. What is the main indication for panoramic radiographs?

13. What is a tomographic "slice" or "cut?"

14. Why are panoramic radiographs not recommended for caries detection and periodontal bone evaluation?

15. Is digital imaging available for panoramic units? If so, explain the basic principles involved.

III. MATCHING

Match the items in *Column A* with the appropriate items in *Column B*.

Column A

_____ 1. rare earth elements
_____ 2. tomogram
_____ 3. focal trough
_____ 4. static marks
_____ 5. circular tube motion
_____ 6. thyroid collar
_____ 7. tongue position
_____ 8. patient movement
_____ 9. mandibular condyle
_____ 10. intraoral x-ray source
_____ 11. open and closed view
_____ 12. slouching patient
_____ 13. tomographic series
_____ 14. first panoramic unit
_____ 15. ghost image

Column B

a. plane of acceptable detail
b. TMJ tomography
c. Panorex
d. tightly packed film
e. objects with high density
f. radiopaque triangle
g. seen on pantomograms
h. not used for pantomograms
i. thyroid collar
j. multiple cuts
k. pharyngeal air space
l. rotating anode
m. blurred image
n. intensifying screen
o. laminogram
p. tomogram
q. distorted image

IV. COMPLETE THESE STATEMENTS

1. Three anatomic landmarks seen on panoramic films that do not appear on intraoral full-mouth series are the

   _____,

   _____, and

   _____.

2. The area of the maxilla that is seen with least amount of definition on a panoramic radiograph is the

   _____.

3. The panoramic image does not have the same

   _____ that is seen on intraoral periapical or bitewing images.

4. The main advantage of a panoramic radiograph over intraoral periapical radiographs is the _____.

5. The bilateral radiolucent (RL) structures seen crossing the ramus of the mandible on panoramic radiographs

   are the _____.

6. Multiple black linear streaks on a panoramic radiograph are a result of _____.

7. Another name for the "plane of acceptable detail" is

   the _____.

8. In comparing patient radiation dose, panoramic

   radiographs require _____
   radiation than a full-mouth series.

9. In panoramic radiography, the midsagittal plane

   should be _____ to the

   floor and the _____

   plane and the _____

   line should be _____
   to the floor for correct patient positioning.

10. When the technician is taking a panoramic radiograph, the patient's tongue should always be

    _____.

11. The main disadvantage of panoramic images when compared to a full-mouth survey is _____.

Chapter **12** **Panoramic Radiography**

12. A lead apron should be used without a _____ for panoramic radiography.

13. A recently reported use of panoramic projections is the detection of _____ in the patient's neck region.

14. An image from the other side of the patient's jaw that is seen as a blurred shadow is called a _____ image.

15. The most skilled operator requires at least 15 to 20 minutes to perform an intraoral survey; pantomographs can be taken in less than _____.

V. MULTIPLE CHOICE

Select the best answer.

1. When taking a panoramic radiograph, the patient's lead apron should
   a. be placed in the usual manner
   b. not be used at all
   c. be placed on the back of the patient
   d. not be placed lower than the clavicles
   e. be placed over the thyroid area

2. Object scatter degrading the image is not a concern in panoramic radiography
   a. because of the rotation of the tube head
   b. because of the narrow slit beam
   c. because of the inherent filtration
   d. because the patient is seated
   e. because of the intensifying screens

3. In positioning a patient for panoramic radiography, if the patient's head is tilted up
   a. a right oblique (RO) triangle is seen in the mandibular anterior region
   b. an RL line is seen above the apices of the maxillary teeth
   c. the chin is back and the forehead is forward
   d. the RO palate is superimposed over the apices of the upper teeth
   e. the lower anterior teeth appear narrow and blurred

4. Each successive panoramic image appears lighter than the one before. Which of the following corrections should be made?
   a. increase the mA setting
   b. increase the kVp setting
   c. change the intensifying screen
   d. change the developer solution
   e. reduce the temperature of the developer

5. Which of the following anatomic structures is usually not seen on intraoral periapical radiographs but is seen on pantomograms?
   a. mental foramen
   b. mandibular foramen
   c. mylohyoid ridge
   d. coronoid process
   e. median palatal suture

6. If the lead apron is placed too high on the patient,
   a. it will create a large RL on the resultant image
   b. it will create a large RO on the resultant image
   c. it will create an RO on the maxilla
   d. it will obliterate all the mandibular teeth
   e. it will create a vertical RL line on the resultant image

7. The main reason for taking a panoramic radiograph would be
   a. to lower the patient's exposure
   b. to see the borders of a lesion that are larger than periapical film
   c. that it requires less time
   d. for better object definition
   e. the film cost

8. Grids are usually not used with panoramic units because
   a. there is no object scatter
   b. the moving field size is very narrow
   c. the motion makes grids ineffective
   d. the film is too sensitive
   e. the mA setting is not high enough

9. Panoramic radiographs cannot be used for detection of
   a. impacted teeth
   b. jaw fractures
   c. caries and periodontal disease
   d. large areas of pathology
   e. eruption patterns

10. In taking a tomographic series, the depth of "cuts" can be varied by
    a. varying the focal object distance
    b. changing the kVp setting
    c. varying the mA setting
    d. changing the type of motion
    e. increasing the exposure time

11. The main advantage of using an intraoral source for panoramic radiography is
    a. better tooth definition
    b. less image distortion
    c. no film is necessary
    d. significant reduction in patient radiation dose
    e. less image magnification

12. Common positioning requirements for panoramic units include
    a. the anterior teeth are positioned in the proper groove in the bite block
    b. the ala-tragus line should be parallel to the floor
    c. the midsagittal plane should be perpendicular to the floor
    d. the chin should not be angled up or down
    e. all of the above

13. In positioning the patient for a pantomographic radiograph, if the patient is too far forward
    a. the hard palate will be superimposed on the maxillary anteriors
    b. the upper and lower anterior teeth will be blurred and narrowed
    c. the film cassette will hit the patient's head
    d. the posterior teeth will be blurred
    e. there will be an RL streak on the image

14. The use of rare earth intensifying screens in conventional pantomographic units
    a. is not possible
    b. is not necessary
    c. is recommended
    d. would not decrease the radiation dose to the brain
    e. would not decrease the radiation dose to the thyroid

15. Advantages of panoramic radiography include all of the following *except*
    a. less time
    b. better patient cooperation
    c. overuse
    d. lower bone marrow dose
    e. simple to perform

VI. TRUE/FALSE

Select whether each statement is true (**T**) or false (**F**). Circle the correct answer.

1. A panoramic radiograph is produced by moving the film and x-ray source in the same direction around the patient. **T/F**
2. Most of the errors in panoramic radiography are as a result of poor patient positioning. **T/F**
3. If the patient is positioned too far forward, the lower anterior teeth will appear blurred and widened. **T/F**
4. The main indication for panoramic radiography is attaining a larger field size than is possible with periapical radiography. **T/F**
5. Ghosting will occur if static electricity is caused during processing of panoramic film. **T/F**

VII. ORDERING QUESTIONS

Place the numbers 1, 2, 3, 4, and 5 in the spaces provided below to indicate the proper ordering sequence for the following questions.

1. Place the following common positioning requirements for panoramic units in the order that they should be considered when exposing panoramic radiographs:

    _____ Bite block position

    _____ Chin position

    _____ Head position

    _____ Frankfort plane or ala-tragus line

    _____ Midsagittal plane

2. Put the following rules for panoramic patient preparation and positioning in their recommended order of occurrence (from first to last):

    _____ Seat or stand the patient in the most erect position possible.

    _____ Ask the patient to remove any metallic objects from his or her head and neck region.

    _____ Have the patient remove anything on his or her person that might interfere with the movement of the panoramic unit.

    _____ Make sure that all of the recommended infection control procedures for panoramic imaging is followed.

    _____ Explain the panoramic procedure to the patient.

3. Put the remaining rules for panoramic patient preparation and positioning in their recommended order of occurrence (from first to last):

    _____ Align the patient's head so that the midsagittal plane is perpendicular to the floor.

    _____ Place the patient's chin on the chin rest.

    _____ Drape the front and back of the patient with the lead apron.

    _____ Place the bite stick between the patient's maxillary and mandibular incisors.

    _____ Have the patient close the lips and place the tongue on the roof of the mouth.

13 Extraoral Techniques

EDUCATIONAL OBJECTIVES

After reading Chapter 13 of the textbook and completing this exercise, the student will be able to:
1. Define the key terms listed at the beginning of the chapter.
2. List and explain the two main categories of the indications for use of extraoral projections in dental radiography.
3. Know the equipment that is needed for extraoral projections, in addition to the function of each of them listed. Also, discuss the film-screen combination used in extraoral techniques.
4. Describe the film sensitivity of extraoral film, the handling of these films in the darkroom, and the processing requirements for these films.
5. Discuss extraoral radiographic technique, including:
   - List and describe the six steps to be taken when exposing an extraoral projection for dental radiographic purposes.
   - State the indications for use; the receptor, patient, and central ray positioning; and the exposure settings for each of the extraoral projections mentioned in this chapter.

I. DEFINITIONS

Define/explain the following terms.

1. Cassette _____

_____

2. Cephalometric radiography _____

_____

3. Extraoral projection _____

_____

4. Receptor-holding board _____

_____

5. Grid _____

_____

6. Lateral oblique projection _____

_____

7. Lateral skull projection _____

_____

8. Object scatter _____

_____

9. Submentovertex (SMV) projection _____

_____

10. Waters projection _____

_____

II. COMPREHENSION EXERCISE

1. Describe three clinical indications for using extraoral projections in dentistry.

2. Which extraoral projection is most diagnostic for pathologic conditions of the maxillary sinus? How is this film taken?

3. What type of x-ray unit is used for taking extraoral radiographs?

4. What special precautions must be taken in the darkroom when loading cassettes and processing extraoral films?

5. What are the advantages of using rare earth intensifying screens?

6. What equipment is needed for taking standard extraoral projections?

7. How can you identify the right and left sides of the patient in addition to labeling patient information on extraoral film?

8. Explain how and why the film-screen system is used in extraoral radiography.

9. How can one differentiate the left side of the patient from the right on an extraoral radiograph?

10. How does the use of intensifying screens reduce the exposure needed for radiographs?

11. What six factors should be known for every extraoral projection?

12. If a periapical film of an impacted mandibular third molar cannot be positioned so that the complete root can be seen, what would you do?

13. What is object scatter?

14. What is the lateral oblique projection of the mandible used to survey? Why is this projection ideal for visualizing?

15. Why are grids not necessary in periapical, bitewing, and panoramic radiographs?

16. Why do you need a minimum of a 36-inch target-receptor distance (FFD) for a lateral skull projection?

17. What are the advantages of an extraoral film holder over the patient's holding the cassette?

18. Why are grids used in extraoral projections and not for intraoral film?

19. What does varying mA and kV settings depend on in extraoral radiography?

III. MATCHING

Match the items in *Column A* with the appropriate items in *Column B*.

Column A

_____ 1. grid
_____ 2. lateral skull projection
_____ 3. rigid cassette
_____ 4. thyroid collar
_____ 5. midline fracture of mandible
_____ 6. left and right side
_____ 7. minimum safelight
_____ 8. posteroanterior projection
_____ 9. lateral oblique projection
_____ 10. Waters projection
_____ 11. reduce patient exposure
_____ 12. cephalostat
_____ 13. SMV projection
_____ 14. point of entry
_____ 15. fogged film

Column B

a. fractures of the cheekbone
b. improper safelight
c. processing extraoral film
d. articular disc
e. external auditory meatus
f. extraoral projection
g. head positioning
h. cephalometric
i. posteroanterior projection
j. need lead marker
k. maxillary sinusitis
l. position with forehead and nose against cassette
m. intensifying screens
n. object scatter
o. fractured mandible
p. film packet
q. not used in extraoral radiography

IV. COMPLETE THESE STATEMENTS

1. When comparing radiographic detail, it can be said that

   film-screen combinations produce _____ detail when compared with film alone.

2. Some states have statutes that _____

   or _____ certain members of the dental health team from performing specific extraoral radiographic techniques.

3. Patients who have _____

   or _____ cannot open their mouths and would benefit from an extraoral radiographic series.

4. The extraoral projection that is most diagnostic for the

   maxillary sinus is the _____.

5. The two extraoral projections that are needed to visualize a fracture of the angle of the mandible are

   _____ and _____.

6. Orthodontists would most likely use the _____ for cephalometric measurements.

7. In extraoral radiography, the field size is _____ than in intraoral radiography.

8. The lateral skull projection would not be used to visualize a large mandibular cyst because of _____.

9. The _____ provides a means of localizing changes in a mediolateral direction.

10. Grids are not used in panoramic radiography because

    _____.

11. Extraoral films are processed _____ as intraoral films.

12. The increased FFD utilized in extraoral radiography is necessary to get a sufficiently large

    _____ at the patient's face.

13. In both the lateral skull and posterior anterior projections, the sagittal plane of the patient's skull is _____ to the floor.

14. For the lateral skull projection, the central ray is directed at the _____.

15. The _____ projection is used to visualize the sphenoid and ethmoid sinuses.

V. MULTIPLE CHOICE

Select the best answer.

1. The best extraoral projection for viewing an impacted left mandibular third molar is
   a. submental vertex
   b. posterior anterior
   c. left lateral oblique
   d. lateral skull
   e. right lateral oblique

2. Grids are used to
   a. mark films
   b. reduce background radiation
   c. reduce field size
   d. collimate the x-ray beam
   e. reduce object scatter

3. In extraoral radiography, an increased FFD is necessary to
   a. decrease patient exposure
   b. increase the beam divergence
   c. decrease the beam divergence
   d. increase film quality
   e. decrease image magnification

4. The best way to visualize maxillary sinus pathology using a dental x-ray machine is a
   a. lateral oblique projection
   b. maxillary occlusal projection
   c. posterior anterior projection
   d. transcranial projection
   e. Waters projection

5. In taking a Waters projection, the patient's
   a. head is inclined 15 degrees
   b. nose and chin touch the cassette, mouth open
   c. nose and chin touch the cassette, mouth closed
   d. forehead and nose touch the cassette, mouth open
   e. forehead and chin touch the cassette

6. Extraoral cassettes
   a. may be rigid or flexible
   b. contain intensifying screens
   c. are light tight
   d. are available in varying sizes
   e. are all of the above

7. If all of your extraoral films appear dense and fogged after processing while your intraoral films are satisfactory, the probable cause is
   a. the solutions are too hot
   b. white light exposure in the darkroom
   c. the safelight is too intense
   d. the safelight is too weak
   e. the solutions are exhausted

8. Extraoral films are processed
   a. only with automatic processors
   b. by the time-temperature method
   c. by sight development
   d. with special solutions
   e. with none of the above

9. Holding devices have the advantage
   a. of preventing a fogged film
   b. of standardizing techniques
   c. of preventing patient and film movement
   d. Both a and c are acceptable answers.
   e. Both b and c are acceptable answers.

10. A fractured zygomatic arch can be seen on a(an)
    a. lateral oblique projection
    b. posteroanterior projection
    c. Waters projection
    d. anteroposterior projection
    e. lateral skull projection

11. The major disadvantage of using extraoral projections with screens in dentistry is
    a. the cost of the equipment
    b. problems with processing
    c. an increased radiation dose
    d. decreased definition
    e. operative difficulty

12. The screen film used in extraoral radiography is
    a. more sensitive to light
    b. more sensitive to radiation
    c. equally sensitive to both light and radiation
    d. not changed by light or radiation
    e. None of the above are significant statements.

13. A pathologic condition in the midline of the mandible can best be diagnosed using
    a. a right lateral oblique projection
    b. a lateral skull projection
    c. a left lateral oblique projection
    d. a Waters projection
    e. a posteroanterior projection

14. The lateral oblique projection of the mandible is not diagnostic anterior to the canine because of the superimposition caused by
    a. the mental ridges
    b. the mental eminence
    c. the genial tubercles
    d. the anterior curve of the mandible
    e. the lingual foramen

15. Exposure, mA, and kV settings vary with extraoral radiographs, depending on the
    a. film speed
    b. intensifying screen
    c. size of the patient
    d. None of the above are possible answers.
    e. All of the above are possible answers.

VI. TRUE/FALSE

Select whether each statement is true (**T**) or false (**F**). Circle the correct answer.

1. Some states have statutes that prohibit or limit the dental professional from performing certain extraoral techniques. **T/F**
2. Extraoral screen films are less sensitive to light than are intraoral films. **T/F**
3. The lateral oblique projection of the mandible is used for viewing mandibular third-molar impactions and pathology. **T/F**
4. Waters view of the maxillary sinuses is used for maxillary sinus pathologic conditions and facial fractures of the upper third of the face. **T/F**
5. For the SMV projection, the central ray is directed from beneath the chin at 45° to the cassette. **T/F**

VII. ORDERING QUESTIONS

Place the numbers 1, 2, 3, 4, and 5 in the spaces provided below to indicate the proper ordering sequence for the following questions.

1. Put the following factors that should be known for extraoral projection exposure in the recommended order of their occurrence (from first to last):

   _____ The FFD.

   _____ The point of entry of the x-ray beam

   _____ The clinical indication for use

   _____ The exposure settings

   _____ The relationship of the receptor to the patient

2. Put the following steps in exposing an extraoral radiograph in their order of occurrence (from first to last):

   _____ Explain the procedure to the patient.

   _____ Perform the proper infection control procedures.

   _____ Set the exposure settings.

   _____ Place the receptor in the holding device.

   _____ Position the patient's head properly, align the x-ray beam, and press the exposure button.

3. Put the following indications for use of extraoral projections in the order listed (from first to last):

   _____ To examine large lesions and traumatic conditions in the head and neck region.

   _____ When the patient cannot or will not open the mouth to place intraoral receptors.

   _____ To obtain a larger field size.

   _____ To evaluate growth and development in children.

   _____ To view impacted teeth.

14 Radiography of the Temporomandibular Joint

EDUCATIONAL OBJECTIVES

After reading Chapter 14 of the textbook and completing this exercise, the student will be able to:
1. Define the key terms listed at the beginning of the chapter.
2. Explain why the anatomy of the temporomandibular joint (TMJ) can cause imaging of the area to be difficult, and list the pathologic lesions related to TMJ disorders that can be seen on radiographs.
3. State the clinical indication; receptor, patient, and central ray positioning; and the exposure setting for the transcranial TMJ projection.
4. Describe the use of the submentovertex, panoramic, conventional tomography, computed tomography (CT), and cone beam computed tomography (CBCT) in TMJ dental imaging.
5. Explain the unique role of magnetic resonance imaging (MRI) in dentistry for TMJ evaluation.
6. Define *arthrography,* and explain its use in TMJ dental imaging.

I. DEFINITIONS

Define/explain the following terms.

1. Arthritic changes _____

_____

2. Articular disc _____

_____

3. Arthrography _____

_____

4. Basilar projection _____

_____

5. Computed tomography (CT) _____

_____

6. Contrast medium _____

_____

7. External auditory meatus _____

_____

8. Magnetic resonance imaging (MRI) _____

_____

9. Positioning board _____

_____

10. Transcranial technique _____

_____

II. COMPREHENSION EXERCISE

1. Discuss the use of conventional tomography in TMJ radiography.

2. How is a contrast medium used in articular disc imaging?

3. Which anatomic structures of the TMJ cannot be seen with routine radiographic imaging?

4. List the pathologic conditions of the TMJ that may be visible on radiographs.

5. Why should dental professionals feel comfortable in dealing with radiographic images of the TMJ?

6. Explain the advantage of using CT in TMJ radiography.

7. Briefly describe the transcranial imaging technique used in viewing the TMJ.

8. What is the advantage of using positioning boards in the transcranial imaging technique?

9. Which anatomic structures of the TMJ should be identifiable on radiographs?

10. Why is MRI very effective in viewing the articular disc of the TMJ? Explain.

III. MATCHING

Match the items in *Column A* with the appropriate items in *Column B*.

Column A

_____ 1. CT

_____ 2. articular disc

_____ 3. TMJ pathology

_____ 4. MRI

_____ 5. panoramic radiograph

_____ 6. positioning device

_____ 7. weak signal

_____ 8. strong signal

_____ 9. SMV projection

_____ 10. arthrography

Column B

a. soft-tissue imaging

b. entire maxilla and mandible

c. axial plane

d. meniscus

e. lateral skull projection

f. high density

g. opaque contrast medium

h. ankylosis

i. cephalometric radiograph

j. low density

k. viewing in three planes

l. transcranial technique

IV. COMPLETE THESE STATEMENTS

1. Patients with symptoms relating to the _____ are not uncommon in dental practice.

2. _____ is very effective for viewing the articular disc.

3. In _____ the articular disc is outlined with an opaque contrast medium.

4. CT enables viewing of an area in _____ planes.

5. The _____ projection can also be used as a scout film for tomograms of the TMJ.

6. The internal and external _____ muscles are not seen on radiographs.

7. Since the TMJ is a movable structure, the condyle should be viewed in _____ positions.

8. The joint is anatomically bound laterally by the _____ arch.

9. Before the wide use of CT in TMJ imaging, _____ was used to examine the condyles radiographically.

10. The TMJ is anatomically bound medially by the _____ of the temporal bone.

V. MULTIPLE CHOICE

Select the best answer.

1. Which of the following imaging techniques is considered invasive and may result in related complications?
   a. CT
   b. MRI
   c. SMV projection
   d. arthrography
   e. none of the above

2. Pathology of the TMJ that can be visible on radiographs may include
   a. disc displacement
   b. fibrous adhesions
   c. malignant tumors
   d. a and b only
   e. all of the above

3. The most important reason for using an angling board in transcranial radiography of the TMJ is
   a. it is easier
   b. less radiation is used
   c. open and closed positions can be compared accurately
   d. it saves film
   e. none of the above

4. Of the following, which method is most effective in producing diagnostic images of the articular disc?
   a. MRI
   b. conventional tomography
   c. CT
   d. panoramic radiography
   e. none of the above

5. The cassette used when producing four views of the TMJ is usually a
   a. 5 × 7-inch cassette
   b. 5 × 12-inch cassette
   c. 8 × 13-inch cassette
   d. 8 × 10-inch cassette
   e. none of the above

6. A conventional panoramic radiograph will show both the right and left joints in
   a. the sagittal plane
   b. the frontal plane
   c. the occlusal plane
   d. the lateral plane
   e. all of the above

7. On an MRI of the TMJ, the articular disc will appear
   a. opaque
   b. lucent
   c. mixed
   d. radiopaque
   e. none of the above

8. On a radiograph, the fibrocartilage associated with the TMJ will appear
   a. right oblique
   b. radiolucent
   c. opaque
   d. mixed
   e. none of the above

9. Which structures of the TMJ will appear radiopaque on a radiograph?
   a. the condyles, articular disc, and meniscus
   b. the glenoid fossa, cartilage, and articular fossa
   c. the condyles, neck of the condyles, and articular eminence
   d. the internal and external pterygoid muscles
   e. none of the above

10. In which three positions should the TMJ be viewed?
    a. open, shifted right, and shifted left
    b. closed, shifted right, and shifted left
    c. open, closed, rest
    d. closed, rest, slightly open
    e. none of the above

VI. TRUE/FALSE

Select whether each statement is true (**T**) or false (**F**). Circle the correct answer.

1. Patients with TMJ symptoms are very uncommon in dental practice. **T/F**
2. The articular disc is a minor source of TMJ disorders. **T/F**
3. Some panoramic units have specific programs for the TMJ that will also allow one to take views in the open and closed positions. **T/F**
4. Before the wide use of CT scanning, conventional tomography was one of the better ways to examine the condyle radiographically. **T/F**
5. Arthrography is an invasive procedure that may have complications. **T/F**

VII. ORDERING QUESTIONS

Place the numbers 1, 2, 3, 4, and 5 in the spaces provided below to indicate the proper ordering sequence for the following questions.

1. Put the following factors for the transcranial TMJ projection in the order that they should be considered for this exposure (from first to last):

   _____ Receptor position

   _____ Patient position

   _____ Clinical indication

   _____ Point of entry

   _____ Exposure settings

2. Group the following characteristics of a TMJ imaging technique with the projection they are related to:

Used as a scout film for tomograms
Used as a means of radiographing soft tissue
Is an invasive procedure
Allows visualization of the medial and lateral aspects of the condyle
Used to view the TMJ from the axial plane
Uses a contrast medium

Submentovertex Projection   Arthrography

1. _____   1. _____

2. _____   2. _____

3. _____   3. _____

3. Group the following characteristics of a TMJ imaging technique with the projection they are related to:

Viewing of an area in three planes
An effective means for viewing the articular disc of the TMJ
An effective means for viewing soft tissue
Excellent means for examining the bones of the TMJ
Do not include diagnostic images of the articular disc
Soft tissue appears opaque

Computed Tomography   MRI

1. _____   1. _____

2. _____   2. _____

3. _____   3. _____

15 Digital Imaging

EDUCATIONAL OBJECTIVES

After reading Chapter 15 of the textbook and completing this exercise, the student will be able to:
1. Define the key terms listed at the beginning of the chapter.
2. Discuss the following related to digital imaging:
   - Know the basic elements that are necessary to acquire a digital image.
   - List the three basic types of digital imaging systems and how they differ from each other.
3. State the three types of digital sensors that can be used in digital imaging.
4. Describe the following related to the nature of the image:
   - Define what a pixel is, and explain its role in the formation of a digital image.
   - List the advantages and disadvantages of digital imaging when compared to conventional film-based radiography.
5. State the components of the digital imaging technique and be able to apply them to clinical practice.
6. Discuss the types of digital systems, as well as the legal aspects of digital radiography in dentistry.

I. DEFINITIONS

Define/explain the following terms.

1. Analogue signal _____

_____

2. Charge-coupled device (CCD) _____

_____

3. Complementary metal oxide semiconductor _____

_____

4. Detector _____

_____

5. Digital image _____

_____

6. Digitize _____

_____

7. Direct digital radiography _____

_____

8. Electronic sensor _____

_____

9. Gray level _____

10. Hard copy _____

_____

11. Image manipulation _____

_____

12. Imaging plate _____

_____

13. Optical scanning _____

_____

14. Photostimulable phosphor plate (PSP) _____

_____

15. Pixel _____

_____

16. Storage _____

_____

II. COMPREHENSION EXERCISE

1. What are the advantages of intraoral digital imaging in comparison with film-based radiography?

2. What are the disadvantages of intraoral digital imaging in comparison with film-based radiography?

3. What is the basic concept behind digital radiography? When and by whom was it introduced into dentistry?

4. Explain the difference between direct and indirect digital imaging.

5. Why does digital radiography produce less patient exposure to radiation than film?

6. What are the basic elements necessary to acquire a digital image?

7. Explain the difference between indirect digital radiography and optical scanning.

8. How is image definition measured? How does definition in digital radiography compare to film definition?

9. What are the three basic types of digital imaging systems?

10. What are gray levels?

11. Why is digital radiography described as environmentally friendly?

12. Name the three most common sensors employed in digital radiography. State the basic differences among the three.

13. Can the digital image be manipulated to show a third plane (axial)? If not, why not?

14. What is remote consultation? How does it apply to digital radiography?

15. What advantage of digital radiography is most appealing to dentists? Why?

III. MATCHING

Match the items in *Column A* with the appropriate items in *Column B*.

Column A

_____ 1. RVG (RadioVisioGraphy)

_____ 2. optical scanning

_____ 3. sensor

_____ 4. storage phosphor

_____ 5. digitize

_____ 6. gray levels

_____ 7. digital image definition

_____ 8. image storage

_____ 9. patient exposure

_____ 10. instant image acquisition

_____ 11. digital radiography

_____ 12. pixels

_____ 13. hard copies

_____ 14. image manipulation

Column B

a. laser scan

b. 256

c. processed radiographs

d. computer

e. group D film

f. "filmless radiography"

g. first dental digital unit

h. admissible in court

i. containers for numbers

j. convert to numbers

k. printouts

l. film processing

m. group E film

n. direct digital image

o. 9 to 10 line pairs per millimeter

p. Charge-coupled device (CCD)

q. 60% reduction

IV. COMPLETE THESE STATEMENTS

1. Two types of sensors used in direct digital radiography are _____ and _____.

2. When compared with D-speed film, digital radiography results in an exposure decrease of_____%.

3. When compared with E-speed film, digital radiography results in an exposure decrease of _____%.

4. In the storage phosphor unit, the sensor is scanned by a _____.

5. A digital image is composed of discrete areas called _____.

6. Once acquired, the computer can change the _____ in many ways.

7. The human eye can discern only about _____ gray levels.

8. Digital images can be stored in a _____.

9. Images taken at different times can be placed on the monitor side by side for _____.

10. Digital images can be sent to an insurance company by _____ or by making a _____.

11. In both direct and indirect digital radiography, a _____ is not needed.

12. Because the silver salts found in film emulsion and processing chemicals are not used in digital imaging, there are no _____ and _____ issues.

13. In direct digital radiography, the image appears on the screen _____.

14. In direct digital radiography, the sensor is thicker and more _____ than in indirect digital radiography.

15. The main disadvantage of digital imaging is _____.

V. MULTIPLE CHOICE

Select the best answer.

1. The standard dental x-ray unit
   a. cannot be used for digital radiography
   b. is not capable of producing the short exposure time needed for digital radiography
   c. can be used for digital radiography
   d. is not capable of producing the long exposures needed
   e. is none of the above

2. The storage phosphor sensor is
   a. larger than direct sensors
   b. more rigid than direct sensors
   c. more sensitive than direct sensors
   d. thinner than direct sensors
   e. none of the above

3. The type of digital imaging system that is similar to scanning a document is
   a. direct digital radiography
   b. optically scanned digital radiography
   c. indirect digital radiography
   d. direct digital scanning
   e. indirect digital scanning

4. The human eye can discern about
   a. 9 to 10 gray levels
   b. 256 gray levels
   c. 100 gray levels
   d. 32 gray levels
   e. 100 gray levels

5. Darkroom and processing capability is needed in
   a. direct digital radiography
   b. optical scanning digital radiography
   c. storage phosphor technique
   d. indirect digital radiography
   e. none of the above

6. The most critical part of a digital radiographic system is the
   a. computer
   b. printer
   c. scanner
   d. sensor
   e. software

7. Digital imaging for panoramic units
   a. is now available
   b. cannot be done
   c. is not yet available
   d. increases the patient exposure
   e. needs standard processing

8. A "hard copy" is
   a. a duplicate radiograph
   b. an image that is hard to acquire
   c. a computer printout
   d. a rigid radiograph
   e. none of the above

9. The digital image has
   a. 4 to 8 line pairs per millimeter
   b. 9 to 10 line pairs per millimeter
   c. 12 to 15 line pairs per millimeter
   d. 13 to 16 line pairs per millimeter
   e. 17 to 20 line pairs per millimeter

10. When compared to D-speed film, digital radiography can reduce the patient's exposure by
    a. 60%
    b. 90%
    c. 150%
    d. 200%
    e. none of the above

11. In direct digital radiography, a digital image can be generated in anywhere from
    a. 1 to 3 minutes
    b. 1.5 to 3 minutes
    c. 1 to 4 minutes
    d. 1.5 to 4.5 minutes
    e. 1.5 to 5 minutes

12. The major difficulty in using direct digital radiography is
    a. using the bisecting technique
    b. placing the sensor parallel to the tooth
    c. patient movement
    d. time consumed
    e. radiation exposure

13. Digital images
    a. can be integrated into an office record system
    b. can be enlarged
    c. can be inverted
    d. can be colorized
    e. all of the above

14. Digital intraoral sensors are
    a. autoclavable
    b. extremely sturdy
    c. available in only one size
    d. quite fragile
    e. none of the above

15. All of the digital imaging systems differ in how they
    a. acquire the digital image
    b. transmit the image
    c. display the image
    d. adjust the image
    e. store the image

VI. TRUE/FALSE

Select whether each statement is true (**T**) or false (**F**). Circle the correct answer.

1. The most critical part of a digital radiography system is the sensor that is placed in the patient's mouth. **T/F**
2. A digital image is composed of structurally ordered areas called analogues. **T/F**
3. In a direct digital radiography system, the sensor is connected by a wire to the computer. **T/F**
4. Indirect digital radiography employs the use of storage phosphor plates directly connected to the computer. **T/F**
5. In optically scanned digital radiography systems, regular dental film is used to acquire the image. **T/F**

VII. ORDERING QUESTIONS

Place the numbers 1, 2, 3, 4, and 5 in the spaces provided below to indicate the proper ordering sequence for the following questions.

1. Put the following steps in producing a digital image in the order of their occurrence (from first to last):

   _____ An electronic charge is produced on the sensor.

   _____ An electronic sensor is placed inside the patient's mouth.

   _____ The sensor is exposed to x-radiation.

   _____ The electronic charge is converted to a digital format.

   _____ The image is viewed on a computer monitor.

2. Group the following descriptions in the category (direct or indirect digital radiography) they are related to:

   A laser scanner is used to produce the image.
   The image is seen instantaneously.
   Utilizes PSP sensors.
   The sensors are more comparable to film.
   The sensors can be wired or wireless.
   Utilizes CCD sensors.

Direct Digital Radiography	Indirect Digital Radiography
1. _____	1. _____
2. _____	2. _____
3. _____	3. _____

3. Group the following characteristics as to whether they are advantages or disadvantages of digital radiographic systems:

   Patient education
   Sensor placement
   Fragility of the sensors
   Initial cost
   Reduced radiation exposure
   Image adjustment and manipulation

Advantages	Disadvantages
1. _____	1. _____
2. _____	2. _____
3. _____	3. _____

Advanced Imaging Systems

EDUCATIONAL OBJECTIVES

After reading Chapter 16 of the textbook and completing this exercise, the student will be able to:
1. Define the key terms listed at the beginning of the chapter.
2. Describe the following related to computed tomography (CT) scanning:
   - Explain the procedure for CT scanning.
   - Describe the functions of the axial, coronal, and sagittal planes of the human body.
   - List the advantages and disadvantages of CT scanning.
3. Discuss the following related to cone beam computed tomography (CBCT) imaging in dentistry:
   - Describe the role of CBCT imaging in dentistry.
   - State the process for acquiring the image in the CBCT technique.
   - Discuss the advantage of the CBCT procedure when compared with CT scanning in dental imaging.
   - List the indications for use of CBCT imaging in dentistry.
4. Discuss the mechanism of image acquisition in magnetic resonance imaging (MRI) imaging, as well as the role that MRI imaging plays in dentistry.
5. Define nuclear medicine and discuss its role in medical imaging.

I. DEFINITIONS

Define/explain the following terms.

1. Axial plane _____

   _____

2. Bone window _____

   _____

3. Computed tomography (CT) _____

   _____

4. Cone beam computed tomography (CBCT) _____

   _____

5. DICOM _____

   _____

6. Field of view (FOV) _____

   _____

7. Hounsfield unit (HU) _____

   _____

8. Image acquisition _____

   _____

9. Image reformatting _____

   _____

10. Magnetic field _____

_____

11. Magnetic resonance imaging (MRI) _____

_____

12. Radiofrequency waves _____

_____

13. Signal intensity _____

_____

14. Soft tissue window _____

_____

15. Software _____

_____

II. COMPREHENSION EXERCISE

1. What is the main difference between CT scanning and digital radiography?

2. Explain the advantage of using a CT scan instead of a panoramic projection in the planning for implants.

3. What are the common themes employed between CT scanning and MRI?

4. What are CT numbers? Give an example.

5. Why is MRI a preferred method for imaging the articular disc of the temporomandibular joint (TMJ)?

6. Why has the "A" been dropped in "CAT" scan? What major change in the use of this technique is responsible for the alteration?

7. What is a weak signal?

8. What is the function of the powerful magnet in MRI?

9. Explain how a CT scan could be sent to the referring dentist.

10. What does image reformatting mean?

11. List five advantages of CT scanning in dental imaging.

12. How is tomography used in obtaining a CT scan?

13. Why is there no radiation risk to the patient with MRI?

14. List four disadvantages of CT scanning.

III. MATCHING

Match the items in *Column A* with the appropriate items in *Column B*.

Column A

_____ 1. CT number
_____ 2. sagittal cut
_____ 3. powerful magnet
_____ 4. proton density
_____ 5. strong signal
_____ 6. hard copy
_____ 7. radiofrequency waves
_____ 8. implant program
_____ 9. electronic detectors
_____ 10. information storage
_____ 11. software
_____ 12. weak signal
_____ 13. bone window
_____ 14. water content
_____ 15. zero HU

Column B

a. directs the computer
b. hard tissue
c. HU
d. signals to computer
e. 70% of the human body
f. high density
g. aligns protons
h. soft tissue
i. water
j. computer
k. MRI
l. resonance
m. given to the patient
n. long wavelengths
o. coronal plane
p. reformatted image
q. software

IV. COMPLETE THESE STATEMENTS

1. For proper implant planning using CT scanning, a

   special _____
   is needed.

2. Seventy percent of the human body is

   _____.

3. CT was introduced into radiology in the early

   _____.

4. Radiofrequency waves and x-rays are part of the

   _____.

5. In CT scanning, the _____
   is done in a tomographic mode with the detectors
   traveling 360 degrees around the patient.

6. In CT scanning, the computer collects the x-ray
   beam penetration data in a grid pattern called a

   _____.

7. A black area on an MR image indicates

   _____.

8. A new means to acquire the CT image is a technique

   called _____

   _____

   _____ using a two-dimensional
   x-ray sensor.

9. CT numbers range from _____

   to _____.

10. Because radiofrequency energy waves are

    _____, they cannot cause
    ionization.

V. MULTIPLE CHOICE

Select the best answer.

1. In MRI the powerful magnetic field in which the
   patient is placed
   a. causes ionization of tissue
   b. produces the signal
   c. generates the radiofrequency wave
   d. realigns the tissue protons
   e. does all of the above

2. The CT image can be
   a. displayed on a monitor
   b. stored on a disk
   c. transmitted by phone to other locations
   d. reformatted in other planes
   e. all of the above

3. In CT the image is formed by the
   a. computer
   b. sensor
   c. tube movement
   d. magnetic field
   e. none of the above

4. Fat tissue has an HU value of
   a. +1000
   b. +100
   c. 0
   d. −1000
   e. none of the above

5. The views needed in a CT scan for implant evaluation
   are
   a. panoramic and coronal
   b. coronal
   c. sagittal
   d. axial and cross sectional
   e. all of the above

6. The main application of MRI in dentistry has been
   in imaging
   a. bone density
   b. the maxillary sinus
   c. the articular disc of the TMJ
   d. the mental foramen
   e. none of the above

7. The CT number for water is
   a. 0 HU
   b. +1000 HU
   c. −1000 HU
   d. +117 HU
   e. −50 HU

8. In CT scanning, significant artifacts are produced by
   a. composite restorations
   b. metallic objects
   c. dense bone
   d. static electricity
   e. excessive bending

9. The radiation dose from a head scan is
   a. more than one conventional skull film
   b. the same as one skull film
   c. less than one skull film
   d. not comparable
   e. none of the above

10. The powerful magnetic field in MRI can lethally attract
   a. the operator
   b. the patient
   c. the water molecules
   d. the receptor
   e. any freestanding metal objects

VI. TRUE/FALSE

Select whether each statement is true (**T**) or false (**F**). Circle the correct answer.

1. CT scanning uses ionizing radiation as the energy source. **T/F**
2. Both CT scanning and MRI utilize the tomographic technique in image acquisition. **T/F**
3. Cone beam tomography produces equivalent radiation exposure to the patient when compared to medical CT scanning for dental use. **T/F**
4. MRI utilizes microwave energy as its source. **T/F**
5. Soft tissues have a strong signal intensity on MRI images and appear as black areas. **T/F**

VII. ORDERING QUESTIONS

Place the numbers 1, 2, 3, 4, and 5 in the spaces provided below to indicate the proper ordering sequence for the following questions.

1. Put the following steps for the use of CBCT scanning in dental imaging in order (from first to last):

   _____ Establish the FOV.

   _____ The raw data are three-dimensional, reconstructed, and form DICOM images.

   _____ The CBCT unit takes multiple images of the FOV in a single scan.

   _____ The receptor receives the information generated by the radiation exposure.

   _____ These images are transferred to software and the FOV is viewed in multiple planes.

2. Place the following steps for the use of MRI in dental imaging in order of their occurrence (from first to last):

   _____ The protons release the absorbed energy received by a sensor.

   _____ The patient is placed in a large magnet.

   _____ Radiofrequency waves are applied to the realigned protons.

   _____ The magnetic field temporarily changes the orientation of the patient's protons.

   _____ The information is transmitted to a computer that generates an image.

3. Put the following procedural steps in using radionuclide scanning for dental purposes in their order of occurrence (from first to last):

   _____ The image is recorded by a gamma camera.

   _____ The image is displayed on a cathode ray tube or stored in a computer.

   _____ Radionuclide scans are then useful for examining bone and salivary gland tissue.

   _____ Radioactive compounds are injected into the patient.

   _____ These organ-specific compounds concentrate in the target tissue.

17 Quality Assurance

EDUCATIONAL OBJECTIVES

After reading Chapter 17 of the textbook and completing this exercise, the student will be able to:
1. Define the key terms listed at the beginning of the chapter.
2. Discuss the following related to chairside technique:
   - State the significance of ensuring that all personnel are trained properly and monitored regularly in exhibiting high levels of chairside competence.
   - List the responsibilities that the supportive staff is responsible for in maintaining a sound dental radiographic quality-assurance (QA) program as recommended by the American Academy of Oral and Maxillofacial Radiology (AAOMR).
3. Discuss the following related to conventional radiography quality assurance, processing maintenance, and film maintenance:
   - Describe the QA constituents of monitoring and maintaining the x-ray units in a dental office.
   - Discuss the steps that the dental professional should take in assuring that the processing techniques, equipment, and darkroom are optimally monitored and maintained.
   - Explain the proper storage for dental radiographic film and the importance of checking the expiration date for a box of film.
4. Discuss the following related to extraoral radiography, lead contamination, and digital sensor maintenance:
   - Describe the steps in assuring the proper maintenance of the cassettes and intensifying screens that are used for extraoral radiography.
   - Know the main sources of lead used in dental radiography and the steps in preventing the harmful effects of this substance.
   - Discuss the steps in maintaining the integrity of the digital sensors used in dental imaging.

I. DEFINITIONS

Define/explain the following terms.

1. AAOMR _____

   _____

2. Calibration procedure _____

   _____

3. Certified radiation equipment safety officer (CRESO) _____

   _____

4. Darkroom quality assurance program _____

   _____

5. Lead contamination _____

   _____

6. Lead-lined boxes _____

   _____

7. "Longest in, first out" rule _____

   _____

120

8. Normalizing device _____

_____

9. Quality assurance program _____

_____

10. Reference film _____

_____

11. Step wedge _____

_____

II. COMPREHENSION EXERCISE

1. What comprises the most critical part of the darkroom quality assurance program?

2. List the categories for quality assurance named by the AAOMR.

3. What items should be posted in the exposure and processing rooms?

4. List/explain two ways to check solution strength in a dental office.

5. Discuss the importance of a quality assurance program in the darkroom.

6. How can an office maintain high levels of chairside competence?

7. List the components of an office quality assurance program that would fall into the realm of responsibility of the dental support team.

8. When should the processing solutions be changed? Explain.

9. Discuss a potential source of lead exposure in the dental office that had been identified in the past.

10. What quality assurance steps are taken regarding digital radiography?

III. MATCHING

Match the items in *Column A* with the appropriate items in *Column B*.

Column A

_____ 1. health physicist
_____ 2. automatic processor
_____ 3. step wedge
_____ 4. optimal darkroom conditions
_____ 5. processing solutions
_____ 6. AAOMR
_____ 7. posting current charts
_____ 8. full fixer strength
_____ 9. monitoring of the x-ray generator
_____ 10. reference film

Column B

a. strength of the solutions
b. governmental agency
c. outlined preventive procedures
d. inspection
e. films clear in 2 to 3 minutes
f. density too dark
g. darkroom schedules
h. cleaned weekly
i. predetermined density
j. solutions are too warm
k. films clear in 4 to 5 minutes
l. changed every 2 to 3 weeks
m. checks for adequate safelighting

IV. COMPLETE THESE STATEMENTS

1. In the dental office, checks for processing solution strength and levels should be performed

   _____.

2. The dental staff should check the safelighting and

   light tightness _____
   depending on the workload.

3. An easy way to check solution strength in a dental

   office is by comparison with a _____

   or _____ film.

4. The strength of the fixer can be gauged by noting the

   _____ films.

5. The dental _____ or

   _____ is most likely to
   be the person in a dental office that takes most of the
   radiographs; however, peer review also applies to the

   _____.

6. _____ is a plan of
   action to ensure that the x-ray images will be of the
   highest quality and there will be minimal exposure to
   the patients.

7. In the past, unexposed film was kept in the operatory

   in _____ boxes.

8. Solutions should be stored in a _____
   location in the dental office.

9. A lessening of film density on a processed film indi-

   cates a _____ solution
   and signals the need for a change.

10. The "_____" should
    be followed at all times in an attempt to evaluate the
    chairside radiographic techniques being employed in
    a dental office.

V. MULTIPLE CHOICE

Select the best answer.

1. Part of the quality assurance program includes maintaining the conditions of protective devices such as
   a. thyroid collars
   b. film holders
   c. lead aprons
   d. barriers
   e. All of the above are possible answers.

2. The most critical part of a darkroom quality assurance
   program is
   a. keeping a log book
   b. monitoring the chemical strength and level of the
      processing solutions
   c. monitoring the condition of the film hangers and clips
   d. recording darkroom maintenance schedules
   e. None of the above apply.

123

3. Processing solutions should be changed
   a. once a month
   b. twice a week
   c. every 2 to 3 weeks depending on usage
   d. at least weekly
   e. daily

4. A scientifically controlled way to test the strength of the processing solutions is by use of
   a. a reference film
   b. a step wedge
   c. the coin test
   d. the time-temperature method
   e. the hot processing technique

5. If clearing of a film requires more than 4 minutes, the fixer
   a. is too concentrated
   b. is too strong
   c. is acceptable for use
   d. will be fine after one week
   e. is too weak

6. Unexposed films should be stored at
   a. temperatures of 50 to 70° F and 40 to 60 percent relative humidity
   b. temperatures of 40 to 50° F and 30 to 40 percent relative humidity
   c. temperatures of 60 to 80° F and 0 to 70 percent relative humidity
   d. temperatures of 30 to 40° F and 50 to 60 percent relative humidity
   e. none of the above

7. The lead used to line the lead-lined boxes may oxidize and produce a white lead powder that is about
   a. 40% lead
   b. 70% lead
   c. 10% lead
   d. 50% lead
   e. 80% lead

8. For a darkroom quality assurance program to be effective
   a. the darkroom must be large enough to accommodate the staff
   b. the darkroom should be used for storage of film
   c. the viewbox in the darkroom should not be used
   d. the darkroom must be a darkroom and nothing else
   e. the thermometer does not have to be accurate

9. In order to use films before their expiration date, one should use
   a. the rule of "Selection Criteria"
   b. the "Criteria for Intraoral Radiographs"
   c. the "longest in, first out" rule
   d. the "maximum permissible dose"
   e. the "inverse square law"

10. It usually follows that developer and fixer solutions will need changing
    a. 1 week apart
    b. at the same time
    c. 2 to 3 weeks apart
    d. 2 days apart
    e. too often to perform the task at the same time

VI. TRUE/FALSE

Select whether each statement is true (**T**) or false (**F**). Circle the correct answer.

1. An effective quality assurance policy that monitors the use of x-radiation in a dental office is the sole responsibility of the dentist. **T/F**
2. Maintaining high levels of chairside competence is the basis of any successful quality assurance program. **T/F**
3. The acronym "CRESO" stands for a certified radiation equipment safety officer. **T/F**
4. The chemical strength and level of solutions in both manual tanks and automatic processors must be monitored on a weekly basis. **T/F**
5. Unexposed and unprocessed films, as well as solutions, should be stored in a cold, humid location. **T/F**

VII. ORDERING QUESTIONS

Place the numbers 1, 2, 3, 4, and 5 in the spaces provided below to indicate the proper ordering sequence for the following questions.

1. Put the following components of a well-designed quality assurance program as listed by the AAOMR in order (from first to last):

   _____ Regular monitoring and testing of processing chemicals.

   _____ Regular monitoring and testing of films, digital sensors, cassettes, intensifying screens, and grids.

   _____ Regular monitoring and testing of processing equipment.

   _____ Regular monitoring and testing of chairside techniques.

   _____ Regular monitoring and testing of x-ray units.

2. Put the following components of a quality assurance protocol regarding direct digital sensor maintenance in order (from first to last):

   _____ The operator should not roll over the sensor cable.

   _____ The sensor cable should not be clamped with a hemostat.

_____ The sensor cable should be gently coiled and placed in a protective case after use.

_____ The sensor cable should be carefully uncoiled and all tangles and bends in the cable removed.

_____ The sensor should be covered with a barrier sheath before use.

3. Place the following steps in a quality assurance program involving extraoral radiography in order (from first to last):

_____ Intensifying screens should be checked for scratches.

_____ Screens and cassettes should be checked and maintained on a regular schedule.

_____ Intensifying screens should be cleaned with appropriate solutions at least once a month.

_____ The dental staff member should apply an antistatic solution to the screens.

_____ If an intensifying screen is scratched, it must be replaced.

18 Patient Management and Special Problems

EDUCATIONAL OBJECTIVES

After reading Chapter 18 of the textbook and completing this exercise, the student will be able to:

1. Define the key terms listed at the beginning of the chapter.
2. Describe the general management techniques that a dental radiographer can employ while taking radiographs on patients.
3. Discuss the following related to treating patients with disabilities and special needs:
   - List the steps that the dental professional can take in treating a patient with mobility issues, including those who are wheelchair bound, in the hospital, homebound, bedridden, or in long-term care facilities.
   - Discuss some of the common developmental disabilities that dental professionals may encounter in the dental office and what technique adjustments are required in order to treat these patients.
   - Discuss the modifications necessary when exposing radiographs on patients that are hearing or vision impaired.
4. Describe the techniques that are useful for managing pediatric patients in dental radiography.
5. List the areas in the oral cavity that can trigger the gag reflex and the various management techniques used to help the hypersensitive patient control this body defense mechanism.
6. List the localization techniques used in dental radiography and describe the clinical application for each technique.
7. Discuss the remedies that can be utilized when attempting to radiograph third molars; teeth undergoing endodontic treatment; and patients with anatomic constraints, such as tori, trismus, a narrow arch, or a shallow palate.

I. DEFINITIONS

Define/explain the following terms.

1. Arthrography _____

   _____

2. Buccal object rule _____

   _____

3. Developmental disability _____

   _____

4. Gag reflex _____

   _____

5. Localization by definition _____

   _____

6. Marking grid _____

   _____

7. Maxillary torus _____

   _____

8. Measuring grid _____

   _____

126

9. Radiopaque media _____

_____

10. Reverse bitewing _____

_____

11. Right-angle occlusal projection _____

_____

12. Sialography _____

_____

13. "Same lingual, opposite buccal" (SLOB) rule _____

_____

14. Trismus _____

_____

15. Tube shift _____

_____

II. COMPREHENSION EXERCISE

1. Explain the role of the dental professional in patient management.

2. Describe infection control procedures in dental radiography of which the dental professional should be aware.

3. How has greeting a patient in the waiting room changed since the Health Insurance Portability and Accountability Act legislation was initiated?

4. How can the dental professional convey a feeling of confidence to the patient?

5. What should a dental radiographer do when a patient refuses to have radiographs taken?

6. What will determine how the disabled patient is managed in the dental office?

7. Why is it important for the dental professional to be able to discuss radiation safety with the patient?

8. List and briefly describe some methods that may be used to prevent gagging.

9. What can the dental professional do if the pediatric patient does not cooperate while trying to take bitewing radiographs?

10. Describe three methods that can be used to localize an impaction.

11. What is the proper film order when taking a full-mouth radiographic survey? Why?

12. What techniques can the operator employ to facilitate placement of the mandibular anterior film when the lingual frenulum presents an anatomic constraint?

13. What are some clinical situations that may make it impossible to take intraoral radiographs?

14. List some methods that might be used to introduce a child to the use of dental x-rays.

15. Explain the use of the SLOB rule in the tube shift localization technique.

III. MATCHING

Match the items in *Column A* with the appropriate items in *Column B*.

Column A

_____ 1. "show and tell"
_____ 2. radiopaque media
_____ 3. definition evaluation
_____ 4. arthrography
_____ 5. shallow palate
_____ 6. SLOB
_____ 7. reverse bitewing
_____ 8. right-angle occlusal
_____ 9. low palatal vault
_____ 10. gagging
_____ 11. grid
_____ 12. canine overlap
_____ 13. rubber dam
_____ 14. narrow arch
_____ 15. lingual frenulum

Column B

a. buccal object rule
b. lateral oblique
c. horizontal angulation
d. defensive reflex
e. change the film size
f. superimposed structures
g. temporomandibular joint (TMJ)
h. bisecting angle technique
i. gagging
j. sialogram
k. increased vertical angulation
l. tongue tied
m. pediatric curiosity
n. endodontic radiographs
o. topographic occlusal
p. localization
q. marking

IV. COMPLETE THESE STATEMENTS

1. In localization by definition, the object that is closest to the film has the better _____.

2. In taking a full-mouth series, one should always start with the _____.

3. _____ is a valuable tool in helping dental hygienists and assistants perform their chairside duties.

4. Suggestion, manner, and operator confidence are ways to prevent _____.

5. To overcome maxillary cuspid overlap, the angulation is altered _____.

6. One of the important roles of the dental professional is to try to _____ the patient so that the procedures will be easier for everyone involved, including the patient.

7. Magnetic resonance imaging is particularly useful in dentistry in diagnosing pathologic processes of the _____.

8. In endodontic radiography, it is recommended that the rubber dam be _____.

9. If a disabled patient is completely unmanageable, radiographs may have to be taken with the patient under _____ or _____.

10. Soft tissue can be visualized or outlined on standard radiographs with the use of _____.

11. Hand washing and gloving should always be done _____ of the patient.

12. The obvious challenge in treating the hearing-impaired patient is _____.

13. Two clinical situations where it may be impossible to take intraoral radiographs are _____ and _____.

14. Two methods that may be used to prevent patient gagging are _____ and

_____.

15. Less than _____ % of dental patients have an impossibly sensitive gag reflex, causing radiographic procedures to be completely intolerable.

V. MULTIPLE CHOICE

Select the best answer.

1. The gag reflex is
   a. an acquired habit
   b. not present in all patients
   c. a body defense mechanism
   d. a contraindication for intraoral radiography
   e. a reaction the operator can ignore

2. When a patient consistently moves the bitewing packet with the tongue and bites the packet, the operator should
   a. force the packet into position
   b. scold the patient
   c. hold the packet
   d. do a reverse bitewing
   e. take no bitewings

3. Dental professionals should never
   a. use localization techniques
   b. hold the film in a patient's mouth
   c. change the size of the film used
   d. use the bisecting technique
   e. explain the importance of dental radiographs to the patient

4. Proper patient management is the responsibility of the
   a. dentist
   b. hygienist
   c. dental assistant
   d. office manager
   e. all of the above

5. If an impacted third molar moves mesially on the second film when the horizontal angulation is increased distally, the impaction must be
   a. buccal
   b. on the crest of the ridge
   c. lingual
   d. horizontal
   e. vertical

6. The use of patient psychology to manage dental patients includes
   a. scheduling appointments
   b. screening telephone calls
   c. chairside responsibilities
   d. collecting fees
   e. all of the above

7. A shallow palate that will not allow proper placement of the film for the paralleling method
   a. is found very often
   b. never occurs
   c. is occasionally found
   d. requires that a panoramic film be taken
   e. requires that an occlusal film be taken

8. The lingual frenulum may
   a. present problems in radiographing the maxillary anteriors
   b. make it difficult to place the film parallel to the tooth
   c. prevent the bisecting method from being used
   d. not affect radiographic technique
   e. none of the above

9. Possible dental patient disabilities include all of the following *except*
   a. prominent mandibular tori
   b. hearing impairment
   c. physical disability
   d. vision impairment
   e. developmental disability

10. An impacted mandibular molar can be localized radiographically in the anterior posterior and superior inferior planes by taking
    a. a periapical film
    b. a panoramic film
    c. a lateral oblique film
    d. all of the above
    e. none of the above

11. Gagging in many cases can be controlled or prevented by
    a. general anesthesia
    b. use of undiluted mouthwash
    c. local anesthesia injection
    d. slower technique
    e. all of the above

12. In which dental specialty is the marking grid usually employed?
    a. prosthodontics
    b. periodontics
    c. pediatric dentistry
    d. orthodontics
    e. endodontics

13. In taking mandibular premolar periapical films, mandibular tori
    a. present severe problems using the paralleling method
    b. have no effect on the paralleling method
    c. restrict intraoral radiography to occlusal films
    d. necessitate the use of panoramic technique
    e. none of the above

14. Which of the following is probably the *least* reliable way to localize an impaction in the buccolingual plane?
    a. localization by definition
    b. maxillary right-angle occlusal
    c. right-angle mandibular occlusal
    d. buccal object rule
    e. none of the above

15. Sialography involves injecting radiopaque material into
    a. maxillary tori
    b. salivary glands and ducts
    c. the lingual frenulum
    d. the TMJ
    e. the ventral surface of the tongue

VI. TRUE/FALSE

Select whether each statement is true (**T**) or false (**F**). Circle the correct answer.

1. Patients must feel comfortable and confident about the dental professional's ability to perform the radiographic examination. **T/F**
2. Panoramic radiographs are useful with wheelchair-bound patients. **T/F**
3. Of all the problems one may encounter in intraoral radiography, gagging is probably the least troublesome. **T/F**
4. Structures that lie further from the x-ray film have better radiographic definition than those that lie closer to the film. **T/F**
5. The shallow palatal vault represents a problem in the paralleling technique. **T/F**

VII. ORDERING QUESTIONS

Place the numbers 1, 2, 3, 4, and 5 in the spaces provided below to indicate the proper ordering sequence for the following questions.

1. Put the following steps for the reverse bitewing technique in order (from first to last):

   _____ The film packed is placed on the cheek side of the teeth in the buccal sulcus.

   _____ The radiographer can position the film packet as the patient closes without being bitten.

   _____ The child bites on the tab to hold the film packet in place.

   _____ The x-ray beam is directed extra-orally from under the opposite side of the mandible.

   _____ The resulting film will not have the detail of an intraoral bitewing but can be a useful substitute.

2. List the following suggested management techniques for a patient with a hypersensitive gag reflex in order (from first to last):

   _____ Film order and technique

   _____ Deep breathing

   _____ Lozenges and sprays

   _____ Hypnosis

   _____ Attitude

3. Place the following steps recommended for the tube shift localization technique in order (from first to last):

   _____ All factors remain the same for the second exposure.

   _____ The tube is shifted horizontally approximately 20 degrees mesially or distally.

   _____ It is used to determine the buccolingual relationship between two structures that appear superimposed.

   _____ The two radiographs are compared.

   _____ The SLOB rule is used to determine if a structure is situated toward the buccal or lingual surface.

EDUCATIONAL OBJECTIVES

After reading Chapter 19 of the textbook and completing this exercise, the student will be able to:
1. Define the key terms listed at the beginning of the chapter.
2. Discuss the types of descriptive terminology used in radiography, including how the density of a structure determines its radiographic appearance.
3. Discuss the following related to mounting procedures:
   - State the advantage of mounting radiographs.
   - List the two techniques in mounting conventional films and state which is the preferred method.
   - List the two modes of mounting techniques that can be employed when utilizing a digital radiographic system.
   - List five helpful hints that can be used in mounting radiographs.
4. Describe the following related to radiographic tooth anatomy:
   - Know the radiographic appearance of the components of the tooth and surrounding bone and soft tissue structures.
   - Identify and describe the anatomic landmarks of the maxilla on radiographic images.
   - Identify and describe the anatomic landmarks of the mandible on radiographic images.
5. Identify common restorations on radiographic images.
6. Identify the anatomic landmarks on occlusal, panoramic, and other extraoral images.

I. DEFINITIONS

Define/explain the following terms.

1. Curve of Spee _____

_____

2. Foramen _____

_____

3. Labial mounting _____

_____

4. Lingual mounting _____

_____

5. Orientation dot _____

_____

6. Radiographic anatomy _____

_____

7. Radiographic mount _____

_____

8. Radiolucent _____

_____

9. Radiopaque _____

_____

10. Sinus _____

_____

II. COMPREHENSION EXERCISE

1. What determines whether an object or structure will be radiolucent or radiopaque?

2. Explain how to differentiate between a maxillary premolar projection and a mandibular premolar projection.

3. How does the orientation dot help to mount films in their correct anatomic position?

4. Which is the most radiopaque of all tooth structures?

5. Which is the most radiolucent of all tooth structures?

6. Why does the dental professional require a basic knowledge of radiographic anatomy in order to mount images correctly?

7. Radiographically, how can one differentiate mandibular molar edentulous images from maxillary molar edentulous images?

8. How and why do the lips, cheek, and tongue affect a radiograph?

9. What should be labeled on the mount to establish patient ownership of the radiographs?

10. On which extraoral projections can the maxillary sinus be seen? Which is the best view for visualizing the maxillary sinus?

11. On what intraoral projection is the coronoid process of the mandible seen?

12. How are bitewings mounted correctly?

13. Why is the mental foramen seen as a radiolucency?

14. Does the maxilla or the mandible have a denser trabecular pattern of bone? What is the clinical significance of this?

15. How can the dental professional distinguish between a foramen and a periapical pathologic process by means of radiographic interpretation alone?

III. MATCHING

Match the items in *Column A* with the appropriate items in *Column B.*

Column A

_____ 1. coronoid process
_____ 2. internal oblique ridge
_____ 3. lingual mounting
_____ 4. nasopalatine foramen
_____ 5. mandibular foramen
_____ 6. curve of Spee
_____ 7. labial mounting
_____ 8. cementum
_____ 9. zygomatic process of maxilla
_____ 10. nutrient canals
_____ 11. enamel
_____ 12. illuminator
_____ 13. greater radiation penetration
_____ 14. mental foramen
_____ 15. genial tubercle

Column B

a. vertical radiolucent lines
b. viewbox
c. lower incisor projection
d. most radiopaque tooth structures
e. radiopaque covering on the root
f. not seen on a periapical survey
g. maxillary molar projection
h. patient's right on viewer's left
i. mylohyoid ridge
j. mandibular condyle
k. U-shaped radiopacity
l. lower premolar projection
m. maxillary incisor projection
n. patient's left on viewer's left
o. radiolucent
p. bitewing radiographs
q. radiopaque band

IV. COMPLETE THESE STATEMENTS

1. The most universally accepted way to mount radiographs is the _____ method.

2. The mandibular canal can usually be seen on the _____ and periapical _____ radiographs.

3. When mounting radiographs, it is important to remember that most roots curve _____.

4. The mental foramen, when it is superimposed on the apex of the premolar, can resemble _____ _____.

5. The most radiopaque of all tooth structures is _____.

6. Cancellous bone radiographically is composed of small radiolucent compartments known as _____ separated by a radiopaque honeycomb pattern called _____ _____.

7. A cement base under a deep restoration will appear _____ on a radiograph.

8. An acrylic crown will appear _____ _____ on a radiograph.

9. The _____ is a depression in the labial plate in the maxillary lateral incisor area.

10. The nasal cavity may be seen on a _____ _____ and a _____ _____ periapical radiograph.

11. Roots of the maxillary molars can seem to be in the _____ when seen on radiographs.

12. The _____ is seen as a radiolucent area below the mylohyoid ridge.

13. Maxillary premolars usually have _____ root(s) whereas mandibular premolars have

_____ root(s).

14. Metallic restorations will appear _____ on radiographs.

15. When interpreting occlusal films, the dental professional must remember that the projection is in the

_____ plane.

V. MULTIPLE CHOICE

1. The periodontal ligament surrounding a normal tooth appears radiographically as
   a. an unbroken radiopaque line around the tooth's root
   b. a radiopaque line on the lateral sides of the root
   c. an unbroken radiolucent line around the tooth's root
   d. a radiolucent line around the apical portion only
   e. an unbroken radiolucent outline around the crown and root

2. Which of the following structures appear radiolucent on a radiograph?
   a. nares, median suture, medullary spaces
   b. incisive canal, genial tubercles, nasal fossa
   c. maxillary sinus, mylohyoid ridge, mental foramen
   d. hamular process, nutrient canals, nasal cartilage
   e. coronoid process, mandibular canal, maxillary septum

3. Which of the following is a major part of the tooth structure, appears radiopaque on radiographs, and is seen in both the crown and roots of the teeth?
   a. enamel
   b. cementum
   c. lamina dura
   d. dentin
   e. pulp

4. Which of the following anatomic structures is usually not demonstrated on intraoral periapical radiographs?
   a. mental foramen
   b. mylohyoid ridge
   c. coronoid process
   d. mandibular foramen
   e. median palatine suture

5. Arrange the following in order of increasing radiopacity
   a. dentin
   b. enamel
   c. amalgam
   d. zinc oxide–eugenol
   e. pulp
      (1) c, b, a, e, d
      (2) d, e, c, a, b
      (3) e, a, b, d, c
      (4) e, d, a, b, c

137

6. All of the following tooth structures appear radiopaque *except*
   a. enamel
   b. periodontal membrane
   c. lamina dura
   d. cementum
   e. dentin

7. Which of the following structures appear radiopaque on a radiograph?
   a. maxillary sinus, genial tubercle, nasal cavity
   b. nasal spine, external oblique ridge, mental foramen
   c. internal oblique ridge, median nasal septum, mental ridge
   d. inferior border of mandible, mental ridge, nares
   e. maxillary tuberosity, nasopalatine foramen, maxillary sinus

8. All of the following may be seen on a mandibular molar projection *except*
   a. the mandibular canal
   b. the inferior border of the mandible
   c. the condyle
   d. the internal oblique ridge
   e. the external oblique ridge

9. The occlusal part of the alveolar bone is referred to as the
   a. trabeculae
   b. lamina dura
   c. alveolar crest
   d. medullary spaces
   e. cancellous bone

10. Which of the following appears radiolucent on a radiograph?
    a. nasal turbinates
    b. nasal floor
    c. nasal septum
    d. nasal cavity
    e. nasal spine

11. All of the following may be seen on a maxillary premolar radiograph *except*
    a. the floor of the nose
    b. the buccinator shadow
    c. the maxillary sinus
    d. the maxillary tuberosity
    e. the zygomatic process of the maxilla

12. The radiolucent anatomic structure seen running vertically between the roots of the maxillary central incisors is the
    a. nasopalatine foramen
    b. incisive foramen
    c. nasal septum
    d. median palatine suture
    e. anterior nasal spine

13. Which of the following structures seen on a panoramic radiograph do not appear on an intraoral full-mouth survey?
    a. the inferior border of the mandible
    b. the maxillary tuberosity
    c. the coronoid process
    d. the hyoid bone
    e. the mandibular canal

14. The bilateral radiolucent band seen crossing the ascending ramus of the mandible on panoramic films represents
    a. the hard palate
    b. the soft palate
    c. the pharyngeal airspace
    d. the nares
    e. the uvula

15. Which of the following can be seen on any mandibular radiograph?
    a. inferior border of the mandible
    b. external oblique ridge
    c. genial tubercles
    d. mental ridges
    e. mandibular canal

VI. TRUE/FALSE

Select whether each statement is true (**T**) or false (**F**). Circle the correct answer.

1. All radiographic structures appear either radiopaque or radiolucent without gradations in each category. **T/F**
2. Not all anatomic landmarks are always demonstrated on every full-mouth survey or individual films. **T/F**
3. It is not difficult to distinguish cementum from dentin on a radiograph. **T/F**
4. Most roots curve mesially. **T/F**
5. Nutrient canals are most easily seen in the mandibular anterior region. **T/F**

VII. ORDERING QUESTIONS

Place the numbers 1, 2, 3, 4, and 5 in the spaces provided below to indicate the proper ordering sequence for the following questions.

1. List the following generalizations that aid in mounting in order (from first to last):

   _____ Maxillary premolars usually have two roots; mandibular premolars have one root.

   _____ Most roots curve distally.

   _____ Look for the curve of Spee while mounting bitewing radiographs.

   _____ Mandibular molars have two roots with interradicular bone visible and maxillary molars have three roots.

_____ The crowns of the maxillary incisor teeth are wider and they also have longer roots than the mandibular incisor teeth.

2. Arrange the following tooth structures in their respective category (Radiolucent or Radiopaque):

Enamel

Medullary spaces

Pulp canal

Pulp chamber

Cementum

Dentin

Periodontal membrane

Lamina dura

Radiopaque   **Radiolucent**

1._____   1. _____

2._____   2. _____

3._____   3. _____

4._____   4. _____

3. Arrange the following anatomic landmarks in their respective category (maxillary landmarks or mandibular landmarks):

Mental foramen

Incisive foramen

Hamulus

Internal oblique ridge

Zygoma

Genial tubercles

Lingual foramen

Inverted "Y"

Maxillary Landmarks   **Mandibular Landmarks**

1._____   1. _____

2._____   2. _____

3._____   3. _____

4._____   4. _____

139

20 Principles of Radiographic Interpretation

I. DEFINITIONS

Define/explain the following terms:

1. Anatomic landmark _____

_____

2. Benign lesion _____

_____

3. Bilateral lesion _____

_____

4. Differential diagnosis _____

_____

5. Interpretation _____

_____

6. Malignant lesion _____

_____

7. Radiolucent image _____

_____

8. Radiopaque image _____

_____

9. Unilateral lesion _____

_____

10. Vitality testing _____

_____

II. COMPREHENSION EXERCISE

1. Why are the borders of a lesion important?

2. What are the three steps to be taken when interpreting dental radiographs?

3. What is considered advanced imaging?

4. Why is it important to the interpretation process for the dental professional to avoid committing technical exposure and processing errors?

5. When should a diagnostician order advanced radiographic studies?

6. Why should the dental professional ask a patient to state his or her chief complaint?

7. What is the importance of previous radiographic images?

8. What is the importance of seeing a suspicious oral lesion on three planes?

9. What is the significance of a lesion that appears bilaterally?

10. Why is it important to visualize dentulous as well as edentulous areas on radiographs?

III. MATCHING

Match the items in *Column A* with the appropriate items in *Column B*.

Column A

_____ 1. edentulous projections
_____ 2. anatomic landmarks
_____ 3. buccal plate intact
_____ 4. horizontal overlap
_____ 5. root resorption
_____ 6. teeth movement
_____ 7. interpretation
_____ 8. distinct borders
_____ 9. median palatine cyst
_____ 10. diagnosis

Column B

a. third-dimension visualization
b. an explanation
c. located in the maxilla
d. identification of disease
e. cyst
f. within normal limits
g. benign lesion
h. faulty operator technique
i. malignancy
j. should be taken
k. advanced imaging
l. periapical radiograph

IV. COMPLETE THESE STATEMENTS

1. Previous films are important because they _____

   _____.

2. To produce adequate diagnostic films, the operator

   should know _____.

3. Most bone lesions are _____.

4. Approximately _____%
   of all pathologic oral conditions are the result of
   nonvital teeth.

5. One must see all of the _____
   of a lesion.

6. _____ are located in
   very specific areas in the oral cavity and are diagnostically within normal limits.

7. Poorly defined borders of a lesion are usually seen in

   _____ lesions.

8. A lesion is considered _____

   if it has one compartment and _____
   if there is more than one compartment.

9. An area that is _____
   should be radiographed in order to examine the area
   for impaction, unerupted teeth, and bone pathologic
   processes.

10. Rapidly growing lesions that do not have distinct

    borders are usually _____
    lesions.

V. MULTIPLE CHOICE

Select the best answer.

1. An example of an anatomic landmark resembling a
   periapical radiolucency (PAR) is the
   a. zygomatic arch
   b. mental foramen
   c. internal oblique ridge
   d. external oblique ridge
   e. anterior nasal spine

2. The interpretation of radiographs primarily provides
   the basis for building a
   a. chief complaint
   b. diagnosis
   c. prevention plan
   d. treatment plan
   e. dental history

3. The patient's chief complaint may be
   a. swelling
   b. pain
   c. loose teeth
   d. bleeding
   e. all of the above

4. Which of the following is *not* a step that is to be taken
   in building a diagnosis?
   a. interpretation of what has been identified
   b. identification of an area or structure that is
      questionable
   c. diagnosis based on the interpretation
   d. extraction of a tooth that is symptomatic
   e. distinguishing an anatomic landmark from a pathologic lesion

5. A dental professional may want to use MRI
   a. for visualizing the articulator disc
   b. for cross-sectional views
   c. for evaluating previous fillings
   d. instead of a panoramic radiograph
   e. to evaluate the overlapping of teeth

6. Dental professionals should develop the skills to
   a. identify all normal anatomy
   b. identify tooth structure
   c. identify bone structure
   d. identify artifacts
   e. do all of the above

7. A rapidly growing, radiolucent lesion with irregular
   borders in the oral cavity could be a sign of
   a. a cyst
   b. an infectious lesion
   c. a devitalized defect
   d. a malignancy
   e. an anatomic landmark

8. Possible pathologic lesions should be described by
   a. size
   b. tooth movement
   c. bone resorption
   d. root resorption
   e. all of the above

9. Most lesions in the oral cavity are
   a. radiopaque
   b. radiolucent
   c. both radiolucent and radiopaque
   d. It depends on whether it is within normal limits or
      not.
   e. There is not enough information given in the reference
      text to answer this question.

10. Other signs and symptoms that can be used in establishing a diagnosis along with radiographic interpretation are
    a. the patient's chief complaint
    b. biopsy
    c. medical history
    d. clinical examination
    e. all of the above

VI. TRUE/FALSE

Select whether each statement is true (**T**) or false (**F**). Circle the correct answer.

1. Interpretation of the radiographs is the only step necessary in formulating a diagnosis. **T/F**
2. To produce adequate diagnostic films, the dental professional must know what relevant information is being sought from the radiograph. **T/F**
3. About 70% of all pathologic conditions seen in the jaws are the result of nonvital teeth and their sequelae. **T/F**
4. Most bilateral findings are normal anatomic landmarks. **T/F**
5. Malignant lesions tend to grow slowly. **T/F**

VII. ORDERING QUESTIONS

Place the numbers 1, 2, 3, 4, and 5 in the spaces provided below to indicate the proper ordering sequence for the following questions.

1. Put the steps in exposing, interpreting, and establishing a diagnosis in their preferred order (from first to last):
    _____ Base diagnosis on the radiographic interpretation.
    _____ Prescribe the required radiographs.
    _____ Interpret what has been identified.
    _____ Expose the prescribed radiographs.
    _____ Identify an area or structure that is questionable.

2. List the following preliminary diagnostic questions in their suggested order (from first to last):
    _____ Have periapical and bitewing radiographs been taken recently?
    _____ What is the patient's chief complaint?
    _____ What were the clinical findings that prompted the dental professional to request the radiographs?
    _____ What radiographic projections are available?
    _____ What additional images should be ordered?

3. List the following questions that follow the preliminary radiographic examination in their suggested order (from first to last):
    _____ What does the vitality test reveal?
    _____ Is the lesion radiolucent, radiopaque, or mixed?
    _____ Where is the lesion located?
    _____ Could the suspected "lesion" be an anatomic landmark?
    _____ Is a bone or soft tissue pathology suspected?

21 Caries and Periodontal Disease

EDUCATIONAL OBJECTIVES

After reading Chapter 21 of the textbook and completing this exercise, the student will be able to:
1. Define the key terms listed at the beginning of the chapter.
2. Discuss the following related to caries:
   - Understand the effect of caries and periodontal disease on the radiographic appearance of teeth and alveolar bone.
   - Recognize caries on radiographs, correlate clinical findings with radiographic findings, differentiate caries from anatomic features and restorative materials, as well as evaluate the extent of the carious lesion.
   - Discuss the limitations of radiographs in caries detection.
   - List and discuss the conditions that resemble caries on dental radiographs.
3. Discuss the following related to periodontal disease:
   - Identify the signs of periodontal disease on radiographs.
   - Recognize the extent of bone loss and identify the associated predisposing factors.
   - Discuss and list the classifications of periodontal disease.

I. DEFINITIONS

Define/explain the following terms.

1. Abrasion _____

2. Advanced caries _____

3. Attrition _____

4. Carious exposure _____

5. Cemento-enamel junction _____

6. Cervical burnout _____

7. Enamel hypoplasia _____

8. Erosion _____

9. Gingivitis _____

145

10. Incipient caries _____

_____

11. Indirect pulp capping _____

_____

12. Interproximal bone loss _____

_____

13. Occlusal caries _____

_____

14. Periodontal disease _____

_____

15. Pulpotomy _____

_____

16. Enamel hypoplasia _____

_____

17. Erosion _____

_____

II. COMPREHENSION EXERCISE

1. Explain the role of the dental professional in dental diagnosis.

2. Give an example of how an error in radiographic technique can lead to a deficient diagnosis.

3. Explain how caries appears on radiographs initially and as it progresses.

4. Why does caries appear radiolucent on radiographs?

5. Name some conditions found on radiographs that might be misinterpreted as caries.

6. What is the best way to detect occlusal caries?

7. Why is it difficult to see buccal or lingual caries on radiographs?

8. Name some predisposing factors to periodontal disease that can be seen on radiographs.

9. What oral conditions are bitewing radiographs especially useful in detecting?

10. Describe the appearance of calculus on radiographs. Is it always seen radiographically?

11. Why are buccal and lingual caries difficult to detect on radiographs?

12. What are the radiographic signs of early periodontal disease?

13. What are the radiographic signs of advanced periodontal disease?

14. What radiographic exposure technique is preferred for identifying periodontal disease radiographically? Explain.

15. Explain the radiographic finding of "cervical burnout."

III. MATCHING

Match the items in *Column A* with the appropriate items in *Column B*.

Column A

_____ 1. periodontal ligament space

_____ 2. resembles periapical pathology

_____ 3. lamina dura

_____ 4. bisecting technique

_____ 5. nonpenetration of photons

_____ 6. calculus

_____ 7. not seen on radiographs

_____ 8. early periodontal disease

_____ 9. radiolucent

_____ 10. advanced periodontal disease

_____ 11. short roots

_____ 12. photons penetrate object

_____ 13. interproximal caries

_____ 14. mistaken for caries

_____ 15. poor way to see caries

Column B

a. radiopaque

b. triangulation

c. bifurcation involvement

d. thin radiolucent line

e. buccal caries

f. cervical burnout

g. gingivitis

h. radiolucent

i. bitewing projection

j. thin radiopaque line

k. panoramic projections

l. etiologic factor for periodontitis

m. dimensional distortion

n. mental foramen

o. poor prognosis

p. acrylic

q. occlusal projection

IV. COMPLETE THESE STATEMENTS

After the following terms, record whether they appear radiopaque (RO) or radiolucent (RL) on radiographs.

1. amalgam filling _____

2. lamina dura _____

3. periodontal ligament space _____

4. old composite restoration _____

5. indirect pulp capping _____

6. caries _____

7. pulp chamber _____

8. mental foramen _____

9. infrabony pocket _____

10. alveolar bone _____

11. porcelain crown _____

12. pulp canal _____

13. cement base under filling _____

14. cervical abrasion _____

15. calculus _____

V. MULTIPLE CHOICE

Select the best answer.

1. The best intraoral radiographic projection for detecting caries is
   a. the bitewing
   b. periapical using the paralleling technique
   c. panoramic
   d. a and b
   e. all of the above

2. Radiographic changes evident in gingivitis include
   a. a widened lamina dura
   b. loss of interdental supporting bone
   c. furcation involvement
   d. both a and b
   e. none of the above

3. The most common reason for taking dental radiographs is the detection of
   a. horizontal bone loss
   b. vertical bone loss
   c. caries
   d. faulty restorations
   e. none of the above

149

4. The most likely diagnosis of an interproximal radiolucency just above the cervical line on a clinically caries-negative tooth is
   a. incipient caries
   b. attrition
   c. erosion
   d. cervical burnout
   e. none of the above

5. It is difficult to visualize buccal caries radiographically because
   a. the x-ray photons do not penetrate
   b. of overlying normal structures
   c. of increased density
   d. of decreased density
   e. none of the above

6. Calcified supragingival calculus on the lingual surfaces of teeth is not seen clearly on a radiograph because
   a. it is more detectable on the buccal surface
   b. of superimposition of tooth structure
   c. it is radiolucent
   d. it is not necessary for periodontal diagnosis
   e. all of the above

7. Gingival recession is not detectable radiographically because
   a. the angulation is wrong
   b. soft tissue is not seen
   c. the recession is out of the field
   d. an increased kVp would be needed
   e. none of the above

8. Cup-shaped bony defects are seen radiographically in
   a. the early stages of periodontal disease
   b. the advanced stages of periodontal disease
   c. the stage of periodontal disease associated with abscesses only
   d. early gingivitis
   e. none of the above

9. When caries invades the dentin from the enamel, it is seen as
   a. a radiopacity
   b. advancing straight toward the pulp
   c. spreading laterally and then advancing toward the pulp
   d. calcifying
   e. none of the above

10. As for periodontal prognosis, teeth that have anatomically short roots will
    a. have a poorer prognosis
    b. have a better prognosis
    c. be more resistant
    d. be less resistant
    e. none of the above

11. The infrabony pocket is seen with
    a. horizontal bone loss
    b. gingivitis
    c. poor crown-root ratio
    d. vertical bone loss
    e. none of the above

12. The crown-root ratio as seen on radiographs becomes critical in
    a. caries detection
    b. the choice of amalgam or composite for restorations
    c. designating abutments for a fixed bridge
    d. periodontal probing
    e. none of the above

13. In the clinical setting, caries seen radiographically is almost always
    a. less advanced
    b. missing
    c. further advanced
    d. calcified
    e. none of the above

14. The type of caries best detected on radiographs is
    a. occlusal caries
    b. buccal caries
    c. cervical caries
    d. interproximal caries
    e. none of the above

15. All of the following can resemble caries radiographically *except*
    a. attrition
    b. abrasion
    c. amalgam restorations
    d. composite restorations
    e. none of the above

VI. TRUE/FALSE

Select whether each statement is true (**T**) or false (**F**). Circle the correct answer.

1. Detection of caries is probably the most common reason for taking dental radiographs. **T/F**
2. Incipient caries is not difficult to detect radiographically. **T/F**
3. The first radiographic sign of interproximal caries is a notching of the enamel, usually just below the contact point. **T/F**
4. Evaluating the width of the periodontal ligament space is an important component of a radiographic periodontal examination. **T/F**
5. Triangulation of the periodontal membrane is seen radiographically in the advanced stages of periodontal disease. **T/F**

VII. ORDERING QUESTIONS

Place the numbers 1, 2, 3, 4, and 5 in the spaces provided below to indicate the proper ordering sequence for the following questions.

1. Put the following roles that radiographs serve in the proper diagnosis of periodontal disease in the recommended order (from first to last):

    _____ Radiographs help in evaluating the prognosis of affected teeth.

    _____ Radiographs serve as baseline data and as a means of evaluating post-treatment results.

    _____ Radiographs help in identifying the risk factors for periodontal disease.

    _____ Radiographs help to detect early to moderate bone changes where treatment can preserve the dentition.

    _____ Radiographs serve to locate and approximate the amount of bone loss.

2. List the descriptions of the classifications of periodontal disease, according to the American Dental Association and American Academy of Periodontology, in their correct order (from Case Type I – Case Type IV):

    _____ Advanced periodontitis

    _____ Mild or slight periodontitis

    _____ Gingivitis

    _____ Severe periodontitis

    _____ Moderate periodontitis

3. Place the following conditions that can resemble caries radiographically in the order that they are listed (from first to last):

    _____ Synthetic restorations

    _____ Cervical burnout

    _____ Abrasion, attrition, and erosion

    _____ Enamel hypoplasia

    _____ Pulp capping

22 Pulpal and Periapical Lesions

EDUCATIONAL OBJECTIVES

After reading Chapter 22 of the textbook and completing this exercise, the student will be able to:
1. Define the key terms listed at the beginning of the chapter.
2. Discuss the following related to pulpal lesions:
   - Discuss the role of dental radiographic images in the identification of pulpal lesions.
   - Describe the normal radiographic anatomic features of the pulp chamber and pulp canals, and state the significance of knowing how these normal structures appear radiographically.
   - State the appearance and identifiable characteristics of pulp denticles (or "pulp stones") and pulpitis.
3. Discuss the following related to periapical lesions:
   - Discuss the role of dental radiographic images in the identification of periapical lesions.
   - State the appearance and identifiable characteristics of periapical cysts, periapical granulomas, periapical abscesses, periapical condensing osteitis, residual cysts, residual granulomas, internal resorption, and external resorption.
4. Discuss the three types of cemento-osseous dysplasias (CODs), including how they appear on radiographic images and where they generally appear in the oral cavity in addition to what demographic group is usually affected by these conditions.

I. DEFINITIONS

Define/explain the following terms.

1. Condensing osteitis _____

_____

2. Dentoalveolar abscess _____

_____

3. External resorption _____

_____

4. Florid cemento-osseous dysplasia (FLCOD) _____

_____

5. Focal cemento-osseous dysplasia (FCOD) _____

_____

6. Internal resorption _____

_____

7. Periapical cemental dysplasia (PCD) (periapical cemento-osseous dysplasia [PCOD]) _____

_____

8. Periapical cyst _____

_____

9. Pulp calcification _____

_____

10. Pulp denticle (pulp stone) _____

_____

_____

11. Pulpitis _____

_____

_____

12. Residual cyst _____

_____

_____

13. Residual granuloma _____

_____

_____

14. Root resorption _____

_____

_____

15. Secondary dentin _____

_____

_____

II. COMPREHENSION EXERCISE

1. Explain why vital and nonvital pulp can appear the same on a radiograph.

2. List the causative factors of pulpal necrosis that can be seen on radiographs.

3. List three causes for a change in the normal size and shape of the pulp chamber and canals.

4. What is the first radiographic finding other than etiologic factors of periapical pathology?

5. How can you differentiate between periapical pathology and PCOD (PCD)?

6. What is secondary dentin, and what is its appearance and clinical significance?

7. What are the most common causes for the formation of secondary dentin?

8. How can you differentiate radiographically between internal and external idiopathic root resorption?

9. What tissues are affected by periapical pathology?

10. Describe the radiographic appearance of condensing osteitis. How does it differ from the third stage of PCOD?

11. Why are periapical cysts seen as radiolucencies?

12. In making a diagnosis of a necrotic pulp, why is it essential to see the apex of the tooth on the radiograph?

13. Name some possible causes of root resorption.

14. What are the radiographic signs of pulpitis?

15. Explain the progression of PCOD (PCD) and how it appears radiographically in all three stages.

155

III. MATCHING

Match the items in *Column A* with the appropriate items in *Column B.*

Column A

_____ 1. secondary dentin
_____ 2. condensing osteitis
_____ 3. calcified pulp
_____ 4. root resorption
_____ 5. three-stage lesion
_____ 6. internal resorption
_____ 7. pulp denticle
_____ 8. periapical pathology
_____ 9. fistulous tract
_____ 10. external root resorption
_____ 11. high pulp horns
_____ 12. residual cyst
_____ 13. periapical cyst
_____ 14. pulpitis
_____ 15. decrease in pulp size

Column B

a. seen in young patients
b. pulpal tissue resorbs the dentin
c. vertical bone loss
d. exudate spills from the pulp
e. difficult to see on radiographs
f. pulp stone
g. present in edentulous areas
h. no radiographic sign
i. PCOD (PCD)
j. dentinogenesis imperfecta
k. no treatment indicated
l. radiolucent (RL)
m. idiopathic
n. hard to distinguish
o. agenesis
p. may be asymptomatic
q. chronic infection

IV. COMPLETE THESE STATEMENTS

1. A tooth with a periapical cyst will always pulp test

   _____.

2. PCOD (PCD) has _____
   radiographic stages.

3. _____ periapical
   lesions are always considered in a diagnosis of an intrabony lesion.

4. An apical radiopacity in a nonvital tooth is called

   _____.

5. Marked toothbrush abrasion will cause the pulp to

   _____.

6. _____ appear as
   well-defined radiopacities within the pulp chamber.

7. Radiographically it is difficult, if not impossible, to

   differentiate between the apical lesions of a _____

   and a _____ on a non-
   vital tooth.

8. A chronic periapical abscess may cause _____

   _____.

9. The _____ abscess may
   cause root resorption and a more diffuse radiolucency.

10. To differentiate between a first-stage PCOD
    (PCD) and periapical pathology one should

    _____.

11. To differentiate between a third-stage PCOD
    (PCD) and condensing osteitis one should

    _____.

12. The formation of _____

    _____ may accompany the developmental dis-
    turbance known as dentinogenesis imperfecta.

13. In longstanding internal root resorption, the prognosis

    for the tooth is usually _____

    _____.

14. Periapical pathology is not seen on _____
    radiographs.

15. The most often seen pathologic condition after caries
    and periodontal disease seen radiographically is

    _____ and subsequent

    _____ lesions.

V. MULTIPLE CHOICE

Select the best answer.

1. Which of the following appears radiopaque (RO) on a radiograph?
   a. periapical cyst
   b. periapical granuloma
   c. condensing osteitis
   d. periodontal abscess
   e. none of the above

2. The best radiographic projection for detection of periapical pathology is
   a. bitewing
   b. periapical
   c. panoramic
   d. occlusal
   e. all of the above

3. If a granuloma or cyst that surrounds the apex of a nonvital tooth is not curetted out at the time of extraction, it may
   a. grow
   b. destroy bone
   c. move and possibly devitalize teeth
   d. all of the above
   e. none of the above

4. The radiographic appearance of PCOD (PCD) will be
   a. RO
   b. RL
   c. mixed
   d. all of the above
   e. none of the above

5. An apical radiolucency in a nonvital, asymptomatic tooth is most likely diagnosed as
   a. external root resorption
   b. periapical granuloma
   c. root resorption
   d. condensing osteitis
   e. none of the above

6. Root resorption can be caused by
   a. rapid excessive orthodontic pressure
   b. chronic periapical infection
   c. chronic periodontal infection
   d. all of the above
   e. none of the above

7. The pulp chamber and canals of teeth in older patients tend to be
   a. inflamed
   b. necrotic
   c. calcified
   d. enlarged
   e. none of the above

8. A normal radiographic anatomic landmark that can be misdiagnosed as periapical pathology is the
   a. mandibular foramen
   b. mental foramen
   c. mental ridge
   d. mandibular ridge
   e. none of the above

9. If a maxillary central incisor tests as vital, the most likely interpretation for a radiolucency near its apex is
   a. periapical pathology
   b. maxillary sinus
   c. nasal cavity
   d. nasopalatine foramen
   e. none of the above

10. Condensing osteitis should be treated with
    a. extraction
    b. root canal therapy
    c. no treatment
    d. Both a and b are possible treatment options.
    e. none of the above

11. The density of secondary dentin when compared radiographically to normal dentin is
    a. more dense
    b. less dense
    c. more opaque
    d. the same
    e. none of the above

12. Large high pulp horns are more frequently seen in
    a. young patients
    b. teeth with extensive caries
    c. teeth with deep restorations
    d. abraded teeth
    e. none of the above

13. Which of the following will appear RO on a processed radiograph?
    a. condensing osteitis
    b. sclerotic bone
    c. hypercementosis
    d. all of the above
    e. none of the above

14. Radiographically pulp capping materials will appear
    a. RL
    b. metallic
    c. not at all
    d. RO
    e. none of the above

15. The process occurring when the cells of the periodontal ligament resorb the cementum and dentin of the root is known as
    a. internal resorption
    b. PCD
    c. external resorption
    d. none of the above
    e. all of the above

157

VI. TRUE/FALSE

Select whether each statement is true (**T**) or false (**F**). Circle the correct answer.

1. Most pulpal and periapical lesions are not the sequelae of caries, trauma, intrabony lesions, or advanced periodontal disease. **T/F**
2. The radiographic densities of pulp chambers and canals differ because of size, position in the tooth, and radiographic angulation, but not because of vitality. **T/F**
3. There are no radiographic signs of pulpitis in the pulp chamber. **T/F**
4. It is possible to differentiate between a peripical granuloma and a periapical cyst. **T/F**
5. Periapical condensing osteitis is an RL periapical pathologic condition and should be treated with either root canal therapy or extraction. **T/F**

VII. ORDERING QUESTIONS

Place the numbers 1, 2, 3, 4, and 5 in the spaces provided below to indicate the proper ordering sequence for the following questions.

1. Put the following causative factors of pulpitis in their suggested order of appearance (from first to last):

   _____ Deep restorations

   _____ Pulp exposure

   _____ Tooth fracture

   _____ Previous pulp capping

   _____ Caries

2. Arrange the following radiographic appearances with their respective category (PCOD, FCOD, or FLCOD):

   1st Stage – RL
   2nd Stage – Mixed (RL & RO)
   3rd Stage – RO
   Located in the mandibular anterior region
   Located in the maxilla and mandible in multiple quadrants
   Located distal to the canines in the mandible

PCOD	FCOD	FLCOD
1. _____	1. _____	1. _____
2. _____	2. _____	2. _____
3. _____	3. _____	3. _____
4. _____	4. _____	4. _____

3. Arrange the following radiographic appearances and characteristics of pulpal and periapical lesions with their respective category (periapical condensing osteitis, residual periapical lesions, or root resorption):

   Arose from extracted teeth
   Can be caused by chronic infection or trauma
   Teeth are nonvital
   RO
   RL

Periapical condensing osteitis	Residual periapical lesions	Root resorption
1. _____	1. _____	1. _____
2. _____	2. _____	2. _____

23 Developmental Disturbances of Teeth and Bone

EDUCATIONAL OBJECTIVES

After reading Chapter 23 of the textbook and completing this exercise, the student will be able to:
1. Define the key terms listed at the beginning of the chapter.
2. Understand the formation and radiographic appearance of developmental lesions of the teeth and surrounding bone, as well as recognize developmental lesions of the teeth and bone on dental images and know which radiographic projections are necessary to formulate a diagnosis.

I. DEFINITIONS

Define/explain the following terms.

1. Amelogenesis imperfecta _____

_____

2. Cleft palate _____

_____

3. Concrescence _____

_____

4. Dens invaginatus _____

_____

5. Dentigerous cyst _____

_____

6. Dentinogenesis imperfecta _____

_____

7. Dilaceration _____

_____

8. Enamel pearl _____

_____

9. Eruption time _____

_____

10. Fusion _____

_____

11. Gemination _____

_____

12. Hypercementosis _____

_____

13. Hyperdontia _____

_____

14. Hypodontia _____

_____

15. Impacted tooth _____

_____

II. COMPREHENSION EXERCISE

1. What is a supernumerary tooth and what is its clinical importance?

2. What is the clinical significance of radiographically detecting hypodontia in the secondary dentition?

3. What is the cause of a cleft and where could a cleft occur?

4. Distinguish radiographically between amelogenesis imperfecta and dentinogenesis imperfecta.

5. How can a radiographic examination help in the evaluation of tooth development and eruption?

6. What is a primordial cyst?

7. Describe what teeth would be seen on a mandibular premolar periapical film of a 10-year-old patient.

8. How does an impacted tooth appear radiographically?

9. What are fissural cysts and where are they found?

10. What are the radiographic distinctions between concrescence and fusion?

11. Describe the radiographic appearance of a dilacerated tooth. What is its clinical significance?

12. What are "enamel pearls" (enamelomas) and how are they usually discovered?

13. How does a cleft appear radiographically?

14. What is the best radiographic projection to visualize a median palatal cyst?

15. What is dens invaginatus and how is it formed?

16. Distinguish between a nasopalatine cyst and a globulomaxillary cyst in regard to radiographic appearance and location.

17. Describe the radiographic appearance of a dentigerous cyst.

18. Describe the appearance of a developing tooth follicle.

19. Why is it important to localize impacted teeth in three planes?

20. What are the best radiographic projections to visualize a nasopalatine cyst?

III. MATCHING

Match the items in *Column A* with the appropriate items in *Column B*.

Column A

_____ 1. enamel pearl
_____ 2. fusion
_____ 3. concrescence
_____ 4. dilaceration
_____ 5. nasopalatine cyst
_____ 6. amelogenesis imperfecta
_____ 7. hyperdontia
_____ 8. mixed dentition
_____ 9. taurodontia
_____ 10. hypodontia
_____ 11. cleidocranial dysostosis
_____ 12. dentigerous cyst
_____ 13. hypercementosis
_____ 14. cleft palate
_____ 15. dens invaginatus

Column B

a. normal crown, short roots
b. failure of processes to fuse
c. lack of enamel
d. nonodontogenic
e. supernumerary teeth
f. agenesis
g. enameloma
h. club-shaped root
i. S-shaped root
j. one crown, two canals
k. delayed eruption
l. joined by cementum
m. midline location
n. 6 to 12 years old
o. two crowns, one canal
p. nonvital
q. tooth bud's cystic degeneration
r. dens in dente

IV. COMPLETE THESE STATEMENTS

1. An impacted tooth surrounded by a large radiolucent area is the description of a _____.

2. The condition in which adjoining teeth are connected by cementum is called _____.

3. Periapical radiographs of patients younger than 12 years reveal some evidence of a _____.

4. In Paget's disease of bone, very often the roots of the teeth show _____.

5. The presence of supernumerary teeth is also known as

_____.

163

6. A large symptomatic radiolucent lesion near the apices of vital maxillary incisors is very likely a _____.

7. A buildup of cementum on the root of the tooth is commonly known as _____.

8. The point of invagination in dens invaginatus is usually the _____ of the tooth.

9. The term that describes the condition of congenital absence of many teeth is _____.

10. Dentinogenesis and amelogenesis imperfecta are both _____ disturbances that affect both the primary and secondary dentitions.

V. MULTIPLE CHOICE

Select the best answer.

1. All teeth test vital in an 11-year-old patient. A radiolucency at the apices of a permanent mandibular second molar that has no caries or restorations is probably
   a. a granuloma
   b. a residual cyst
   c. a periapical abscess
   d. incomplete root formation
   e. none of the above

2. Conditions affecting the eruption pattern that can be seen only by radiographic examination include
   a. anodontia
   b. tumors
   c. supernumerary teeth
   d. all of the above
   e. none of the above

3. In dentinogenesis imperfecta, the teeth appear radiographically
   a. with elongated roots
   b. with premature calcification of the pulp chamber
   c. with no enamel
   d. with no dentin
   e. none of the above

4. Most impacted teeth are not visible on
   a. radiographic examination
   b. periapical radiographs
   c. panoramic radiographs
   d. clinical examination
   e. none of the above

5. A fused maxillary central incisor will appear radiographically to have
   a. one pulp chamber, one pulp canal
   b. no pulp chamber, two pulp canals
   c. two pulp chambers, two pulp canals
   d. one pulp chamber, two pulp canals
   e. none of the above

6. Which of the following is not a common supernumerary tooth?
   a. mesiodens
   b. distodens
   c. paramolar
   d. maxillary premolar
   e. none of the above

7. A globulomaxillary cyst will always appear radiographically
   a. apical to the central incisors
   b. distal to the maxillary cuspid
   c. in the midline of the palate
   d. between the maxillary lateral and canine
   e. none of the above

8. The radiographic detection of an enamel pearl on a tooth indicates
   a. nothing clinically
   b. that the tooth may be nonvital
   c. that the tooth should be extracted
   d. that the tooth is a poor abutment tooth
   e. none of the above

9. Teeth with hypercementosis are usually
   a. vital
   b. nonvital
   c. scheduled for extraction
   d. replaced with implants
   e. not treated

10. The best diagnosis for a tooth that appears radiographically to have enamel-like material in the pulp chamber is
    a. amelogenesis imperfecta
    b. fusion
    c. dens invaginatus
    d. concrescence
    e. none of the above

11. The normal range of eruption time for the permanent dentition is
    a. ±9 months
    b. ±2 months
    c. +1 year
    d. ±1 month
    e. none of the above

12. A mesiodens is always
    a. nonvital
    b. found distal to the terminal molar
    c. to be extracted
    d. found in the midline
    e. none of the above

13. A dilacerated root could present a problem when
    a. the tooth should be extracted
    b. the tooth needs root canal therapy
    c. the tooth is endodontically involved
    d. all of the above are possible answers
    e. none of the above

14. A dentigerous cyst should
    a. be surgically removed
    b. be observed every 6 months
    c. be radiographed every year
    d. be radiographed every 2 years
    e. none of the above

15. The best radiographic projection for the detection of an impacted mandibular third molar is
    a. right-angle occlusal
    b. bitewing
    c. panoramic
    d. molar periapical
    e. none of the above

VI. TRUE/FALSE

Select whether each statement is true (**T**) or false (**F**). Circle the correct answer.

1. The developing tooth can be seen at all stages on radiographs. **T/F**
2. If root formation is not complete, a radiolucent area may appear around the root tip. **T/F**
3. Supernumerary teeth, and their relative position to other teeth, are not easily detectable even on the proper radiographs. **T/F**
4. Enamel pearls (enameloma) are small, spherical-shaped pieces of enamel attached to the crowns of teeth. **T/F**
5. Fissural cysts are always found in predictable anatomic locations because they develop along embryonic suture lines. **T/F**

VII. ORDERING QUESTIONS

Place the numbers 1, 2, 3, 4, and 5 in the spaces provided below to indicate the proper ordering sequence for the following questions.

1. Put the following steps in tooth development seen radiographically in their order of occurrence (from first to last):

    _____ Tooth erupts.

    _____ Tooth germ is seen as a round or oval radiolucency.

    _____ The dental papilla appears at the forming apices.

    _____ Crown formation progresses.

    _____ The radiolucent follicle (dental sac) is seen surrounding the crown of the tooth.

2. Arrange the following radiographic appearances and characteristics of amelogenesis imperfecta and dentinogenesis imperfecta in their respective categories:

    Thin enamel of poor quality
    Early calcification of the pulp chambers and canals
    Short roots especially noticeable in the permanent teeth
    Hereditary disturbance
    Dentin and root formation are normal

Amelogenesis imperfecta	Dentinogenesis imperfecta
1. _____	1. _____
2. _____	2. _____
3. _____	3. _____

3. Arrange the following radiographic appearances and characteristics of fusion, gemination, and concrescence in their respective categories:

    Single crown
    Two crowns
    Common root canal
    Joined by the cementum
    Two root canals
    Difficult to differentiate from teeth in close contact

Fusion	Gemination	Concrescence
1. _____	1. _____	1. _____
2. _____	2. _____	2. _____

Bone and Other Lesions

EDUCATIONAL OBJECTIVES

After reading Chapter 24 of the textbook and completing this exercise, the student will be able to:
1. Define the key terms listed at the beginning of the chapter.
2. Utilize descriptive terminology in providing an interpretation of bone and other oral lesions.
3. Discuss the following related to cysts, tumors, and bone lesions:
   - Recognize cysts, tumors, and bone lesions and differentiate their appearance from normal.
   - Understand which radiographic projections are needed to formulate a complete radiographic diagnosis of bone and other oral lesions.
4. Discuss the radiographic appearance of traumatic injuries, foreign bodies and root tips, extraction sockets, salivary stones, exostosis, and enostosis.

I. DEFINITIONS

Define/explain the following terms.

1. Benign tumor _____

   _____

2. Buccal cortex of bone _____

   _____

3. Endostosis (dense bone island, idiopathic osteosclerosis) _____

   _____

4. Exostosis (hyperostosis) _____

   _____

5. Extraction socket _____

   _____

6. Foreign body _____

   _____

7. Fracture _____

   _____

8. Malignancy (malignant lesion) _____

9. Metabolic lesion _____

   _____

10. Mixed lesion _____

    _____

11. Radiolucent (RL) _____

    _____

12. Radiopaque (RO) _____

_____

13. Salivary stones, sialoliths, or salivary calculi _____

_____

14. Trabecular pattern of bone _____

_____

15. Tumor _____

_____

II. COMPREHENSION EXERCISE

1. Name three causes of root resorption.

2. Why is it difficult to identify a root fracture radiographically?

3. How does a bone fracture appear radiographically? Why?

4. How do sialoliths (salivary stones or salivary calculi) appear radiographically? How are they best radiographed?

5. In radiographing tumors, what is the importance of the right-angle occlusal projection?

6. In radiographing tumors and cysts, what is the advantage of using a panoramic projection?

7. How long can an extraction site be radiographically evident and why?

8. What is a hyperostotic line? What is its diagnostic significance?

9. When are foreign bodies most apparent and which are easiest to identify and most commonly occurring?

10. Describe the radiographic appearance of a retained root tip. How can it be differentiated from a dense area of bone?

11. How do metabolic bone lesions manifest themselves? Give three examples of diseases that would manifest in this manner.

12. Would an osteoma appear RO or RL? Why?

13. What is the most obvious radiographic appearance of a malignant lesion in comparison with a benign lesion?

14. Would a cyst appear RO or RL? Why?

15. What two extraoral projections should one expose in a suspected tumor of the maxillary sinus?

III. MATCHING

Match the items in *Column A* with the appropriate items in *Column B*.

Column A

_____ 1. odontoma
_____ 2. malignant
_____ 3. metallic fragment
_____ 4. benign tumor
_____ 5. extraction sockets
_____ 6. fracture
_____ 7. extent of the lesion
_____ 8. parotid gland
_____ 9. retained root tips
_____ 10. dentigerous cyst
_____ 11. mixed lesion
_____ 12. cysts
_____ 13. Paget's disease
_____ 14. ameloblastoma
_____ 15. sialolith

Column B

a. RL
b. lateral oblique projection
c. enlarged marrow spaces
d. cotton wool effect
e. variety of densities
f. mandibular third molar region
g. well-defined lesions
h. density of tooth structure
i. poorly defined borders
j. resembles tooth structure
k. RO
l. associated with impacted teeth
m. see the entire lesion
n. right-angle occlusal projection
o. nonvital teeth
p. evident for up to 6 months
q. RL line

IV. COMPLETE THESE STATEMENTS

1. A sialolith of the submandibular duct can best be seen on a _____ radiographic projection.

2. Salivary stones are a common cause of _____ _____, _____, and _____.

3. An intraosseous tumor that has the density of tooth components is an _____.

4. Three projections for viewing a sialolith in the parotid gland are a _____, _____, and a _____ placed in the mucobuccal fold.

5. Intraosseous malignant tumors will usually _____ the buccal cortex of the jawbones.

6. Retained root tips have the density of _____, making them difficult to differentiate from dense areas of bone.

7. An example of an RO benign tumor is a _____.

8. Only those foreign bodies that are _____ can be seen radiographically.

9. The extraoral projection that is used to visualize the cottonwool appearance in Paget's disease is the _____.

10. Tooth and root fractures can lead to pulp damage and ensuing _____ conditions.

11. The RO line seen on radiographs surrounding a slow-growing tumor is called the _____.

12. In a suspected fracture of the mandible, the two radiographic projections that should be taken are the _____ and the _____.

13. An extraction socket is usually filled in with bone in about _____.

14. A tumor that tends to move teeth is usually _____.

15. An unerupted tooth surrounded by a large RL area is usually the description of a _____.

V. MULTIPLE CHOICE

Select the best answer.

1. Which of the following pathologic conditions appears RO on intraoral radiographs?
   a. a granuloma
   b. a periapical cyst
   c. an osteoma
   d. a connective tissue tumor
   e. none of the above

2. Tumors can appear
   a. RL
   b. RO
   c. mixed
   d. Any of the above is possible.
   e. a and b only

3. The buccal and lingual cortex surrounding a tumor of the mandible can best be seen on a
   a. panoramic radiograph
   b. topographic occlusal film
   c. lateral oblique projection
   d. right-angle occlusal projection
   e. none of the above

4. The radiographic differentiation between a retained root tip and a dense area of bone often can be done by identifying
   a. enamel
   b. cementum
   c. dentin
   d. a pulp canal
   e. none of the above

5. Metabolic radiographic bone lesions can be seen with
   a. Paget's disease
   b. types of anemia
   c. hyperparathyroidism
   d. Any of the above is possible.
   e. none of the above

6. The trabecular pattern of bone in a suspected metabolic lesion can best be interpreted with a(n)
   a. bitewing projection
   b. periapical projection
   c. panoramic projection
   d. extraoral projection
   e. none of the above

7. In making a radiographic diagnosis of a suspected tumor
   a. all the borders of the lesion must be seen
   b. the distal border must be seen
   c. the buccal cortex must be seen
   d. the center of the lesion must be seen
   e. none of the above

8. Extraction sockets are initially seen as
   a. RL areas
   b. RO areas
   c. mixed areas
   d. Any of the above is possible.
   e. a and b only

9. Fractures of the mandible or maxilla may appear radiographically as
   a. an RO line
   b. an RL line
   c. an RL area
   d. a mixed area
   e. none of the above

10. A sialolith in the parotid gland can be seen in a
    a. lateral oblique projection
    b. posteroanterior projection
    c. soft tissue film placed in the mucobuccal fold
    d. computed tomography scan
    e. all of the above

11. When radiographed, all suspected tumors must be viewed
    a. buccally
    b. lingually
    c. occlusally
    d. in all three planes
    e. none of the above

12. On a radiograph an amalgam fragment in an extraction socket will appear
    a. RO
    b. not at all
    c. RL
    d. part RL, part RO
    e. none of the above

13. A common cause of dry mouth, swelling, and pain under the tongue, especially after eating, is a(n)
    a. odontoma
    b. periapical cyst
    c. sialolith
    d. periapical abscess
    e. none of the above

14. Which of the following projections will be diagnostic for the buccal and lingual cortex of the mandible?
    a. panoramic
    b. periapical
    c. lateral oblique
    d. posterior anterior
    e. none of the above

15. The best radiograph for viewing a sialolith in the submandibular gland is
    a. a right-angle mandibular occlusal projection
    b. a topographic mandibular occlusal projection
    c. a topographic maxillary occlusal projection
    d. a right-angle maxillary occlusal projection
    e. none of the above

VI. TRUE/FALSE

Select whether each statement is true (**T**) or false (**F**). Circle the correct answer.

1. Malignancies tend to have poorly defined radiographic borders and destroy normal anatomic structures. **T/F**
2. Many metabolic conditions manifest themselves with changes of the trabecular pattern and lamina dura of bone in the mandible and maxilla. **T/F**
3. Fractures of teeth, especially anterior teeth, are very uncommon. **T/F**
4. Retained root tips do not have the density of tooth structure and are easily distinguished from dense areas of bone. **T/F**
5. Stones in the parotid gland can best be seen on a mandibular occlusal projection. **T/F**

VII. ORDERING QUESTIONS

Place the numbers 1, 2, 3, 4, and 5 in the spaces provided below to indicate the proper ordering sequence for the following questions.

1. Place the steps in describing the radiographic appearance of bone and other lesions in order (from first to last):

   _____ A lesion is discovered on radiographs.

   _____ The dental professional describes the location of the lesion.

   _____ The dental professional establishes the radiographic extent of the lesion.

   _____ The dental professional describes the lesion as RL, RO, or mixed.

   _____ The dental professional observes the borders of the lesion as being defined or irregular.

2. State whether the lesions below are RL, RO, or mixed (RL & RO) on dental radiographic images:

   a. Osteoma: RL, RO, or mixed
   b. Cyst: RL, RO, or mixed
   c. Fracture: RL, RO, or mixed
   d. Root tips: RL, RO, or mixed
   e. Dense bone island: RL, RO, or mixed

3. Group the following radiographic appearance and characteristics of exostosis and endostosis in their respective categories (exostosis or endostosis):

An overgrowth of bone on the surface of the alveolar bone
Appear RO on radiographs

Are identified on radiographic examination only
Are identified on clinical and radiographic examination
Is also known as a "dense bone island" or "idiopathic osteosclerosis"
Internal growths of bone
Most commonly occur on the buccal surfaces of the maxillary canine and molar regions.

Exostosis	Endostosis
1. _____	1. _____
2. _____	2. _____
3. _____	3. _____
4. _____	4. _____

25 Legal Considerations

EDUCATIONAL OBJECTIVES

After reading Chapter 25 of the textbook and completing this exercise, the student will be able to:
1. Define the key terms listed at the beginning of the chapter.
2. Describe and be able to differentiate between state and federal regulations as they pertain to dental radiology and licensure.
3. Discuss risk management, including:
   - Understand the concepts of risk management as they apply to patient relations, ownership and retention of radiographs, and the medical and radiation history.
   - Understand the concept of informed consent.
4. Understand the legal status of insurance forms and the dental records.

I. DEFINITIONS

Define/explain the following terms.

1. Confidentiality _____

   _____

2. Direct supervision _____

   _____

3. General supervision _____

   _____

4. Informed consent _____

   _____

5. Liability _____

   _____

6. Licensure _____

   _____

7. Radiation inspections _____

   _____

8. Respondeat superior _____

   _____

9. Risk management _____

   _____

10. Statute of limitations _____

    _____

II. COMPREHENSION EXERCISE

1. Is it acceptable for the insurance company to request preoperative and postoperative radiographs on a patient? Explain.

2. How long should dental radiographs be kept for a patient after he or she has ceased being a patient in the office?

3. How long does an adult patient have to file a lawsuit after the injury is committed? How long if the patient is a child?

4. Who owns the radiographic series—the patient or the dentist? What rights to the radiographs does the patient have? Explain.

5. What confidentiality issues apply to dental radiographs as a permanent part of a patient's records?

6. Why is it vitally important to keep accurate patient records?

7. What is risk management and who should participate in the program in a dental office?

8. Why is it important for the dental support staff to review the patient's health history before taking radiographs?

9. What is the difference between direct and general supervision in a dental office and how are these principles applied to dental radiography?

10. In what three major categories are the legal considerations regarding the use of ionizing radiation in dentistry included?

III. MATCHING

Match the items in *Column A* with the appropriate items in *Column B.*

Column A

_____ 1. risk management
_____ 2. direct supervision
_____ 3. respondeat superior
_____ 4. negligent
_____ 5. general supervision
_____ 6. full disclosure
_____ 7. informed consent
_____ 8. res gestae
_____ 9. standard of care
_____ 10. Health Insurance Portability and Accountability Act (HIPAA)

Column B

a. "captain of the ship" principle
b. admissions against interest
c. permission granted
d. dentist is physically present
e. at fault
f. confidentiality
g. personal radiation exposure
h. ownership of radiographs
i. dentist can be reached
j. reduce likelihood of suits
k. informing the patient
l. statute of limitations
m. usually performed procedures

175

IV. COMPLETE THESE STATEMENTS

1. The _____ is the guardian of the dental radiographs.

2. The three most important parts of a defense in a malpractice suit are the "_____, _____, and _____."

3. The statute of limitation for an adult patient to file suit is _____ years and for a child it is approximately _____ years after he or she has reached the age of 21.

4. The insurance company cannot request _____ radiographs because their use is considered administrative.

5. All radiographic equipment manufactured or sold after _____ must meet federal regulations.

6. Many states require biannual or triennial _____ of the x-ray machines in the dental office.

7. _____ is the policies and procedures designed to reduce the likelihood of suits for malpractice against dentists.

8. _____, professionally and legally, rests with the dentist and not the dental hygienist or the dental assistant.

9. _____ means that the dentist is physically present in the office when the radiographs are being taken by the dental hygienist or assistant.

10. Radiographs of poor _____ can weaken the defense in a lawsuit for which they are being used as evidence.

V. MULTIPLE CHOICE

Select the best answer.

1. Ownership of the radiographs rests with the
   a. dentist
   b. hygienist
   c. patient
   d. assistant
   e. none of the above

2. Insurance carriers can request
   a. postoperative radiographs
   b. preoperative radiographs
   c. any radiograph taken on the patient
   d. only the patient's radiographs that were taken during the last year
   e. none of the above

3. The dental office supportive staff can participate in obtaining informed consent from the patient, which entails
   a. formulating a diagnosis
   b. formulating a prognosis
   c. explaining the nature and purpose of the procedure to the patient
   d. holding back any information about the procedures to the patient
   e. none of the above

4. The doctrine of respondeat superior is also known as the
   a. res gestae
   b. "captain of the ship" principle
   c. risk management theory
   d. statute of limitations
   e. none of the above

5. The legal considerations with which dental assistants and hygienists should be concerned regarding the dental use of ionizing radiation are
   a. regulations regarding x-ray equipment
   b. risk management
   c. licensure and periodic inspection for users of x-ray equipment
   d. a and b only
   e. all of the above

6. Statements made by anyone at the time of an alleged negligent act are
   a. not admissible as evidence
   b. only admissible as evidence if recorded
   c. only admissible as evidence if repeated
   d. admissible as evidence
   e. none of the above

7. Dental radiographs are considered a part of the patient's dental record and are therefore considered
   a. to be illegal documents
   b. to be negligible documents
   c. to be liable documents
   d. to be legal documents
   e. none of the above

8. If the radiographic evidence presented to the court is illegible, the court may
   a. request the original radiographs
   b. not accept the radiographs as evidence
   c. allow the case to be affected by the lack of evidence
   d. a and b only
   e. all of the above

9. Dental procedures should not be performed without current and diagnostic radiographs because their use is now
   a. the only dental record needed for diagnosis
   b. the standard of care
   c. the only dental record needed for insurance purposes
   d. the only dental record needed to formulate a prognosis
   e. none of the above

10. The patient's records are
    a. discussed freely among dental professionals
    b. discussed only with the dental hygienist
    c. discussed only with the dentist
    d. confidential
    e. none of the above

VI. TRUE/FALSE

Select whether each statement is true (**T**) or false (**F**). Circle the correct answer.

1. All dental x-ray machines either manufactured or sold in the United States after 1974 must meet the federal government's performance standards. **T/F**
2. The dental professional should be knowledgeable about the rules and regulations of the state in which he or she is exposing radiographs. **T/F**
3. Liability, both professionally and legally, rests with all members of the dental staff. **T/F**
4. Dental radiographs are considered part of the patient's dental record but are not considered legal documents. **T/F**
5. The contents or findings in the patient's records are strictly confidential and should never be discussed or shown to anyone outside the dental facility. **T/F**

VII. ORDERING QUESTIONS

Place the numbers 1, 2, 3, 4, and 5 in the spaces provided below to indicate the proper ordering sequence for the following questions.

1. Place the following components of a risk management program in the order listed (from first to last):
   _____ Avoid misunderstandings.
   _____ The patient's records are confidential.
   _____ Obtain informed consent.
   _____ Review the patient's health history and questionnaire and update as necessary.
   _____ Dental radiographs are considered legal documents.
   _____ The dentist is the guardian of dental radiographs.

2. State whether the following HIPAA considerations are components of: 1. Privacy Standards; 2. Patient's Rights; or 3. Administrative Requirements (refer to Box 25-1).

Write the number 1, 2, or 3 next to each of the HIPAA considerations below:

a. HIPAA allows patients to become more aware of the health information privacy they are entitled to.
   a. _____
b. It is recommended that health professionals become appropriately familiar with the law.
   b. _____
c. Covered entities may be given serious civil and criminal penalties for violating HIPAA legislation.
   c. _____
d. A notice of privacy practices.
   d. _____
e. An acknowledgment of receipt notice of privacy practices.
   e. _____
f. Parents of a minor have access to their child's health information.
   f. _____

3. List the following types of legal considerations concerning the use of ionizing radiation in dentistry in their recommended order (from first to last):
   _____ Risk management procedures.
   _____ State regulations regarding x-ray equipment.
   _____ Licensure requirements for dental radiographers.
   _____ Federal regulations regarding x-ray equipment.
   _____ Risk management policies.

Laboratory Workshop Activities

CHAPTER 1

The History of Ionizing Radiation and Basic Principles of X-Ray Generation

1. (Figure 1-1) Label the components in this diagram of an atom.

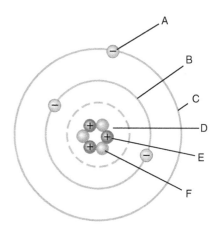

a.

b.

c.

d.

e.

f.

2. (Figure 1-2) Identify the lettered components in this diagram of the dental x-ray tube and list the function of each.

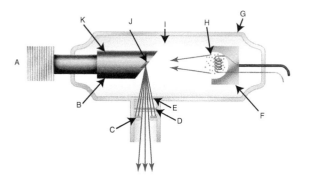

Component	Function
a.	
b.	
c.	
d.	
e.	
f.	
g.	
h.	
i.	
j.	
k.	

3. Provide a schematic drawing of the composition of matter.

5. Draw a diagram of the Bremsstrahlung reaction at the tungsten target.

4. (Figure 1-3) In this schematic drawing of dental x-rays, which x-ray, A or B:

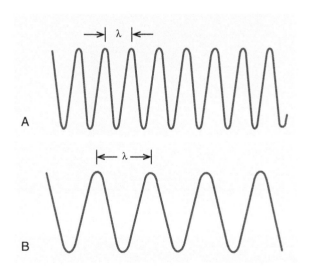

a. has the longest wavelength? _____

b. has the most energy? _____

c. has the higher frequency? _____

d. would be more penetrating? _____

CHAPTER 2

The Dental X-Ray Machine

1. (Figure 2-1) Identify the lettered components in this diagram of the tube head of a dental x-ray machine.

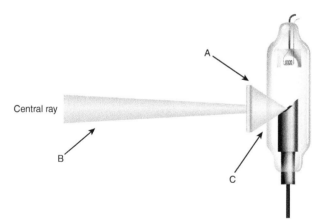

a.

b.

c.

2. (Figure 2-2) Outline in red the areas that would be exposed by the x-ray beam that do not contribute to the image when using circular collimation. Do the same in blue for rectangular collimation.

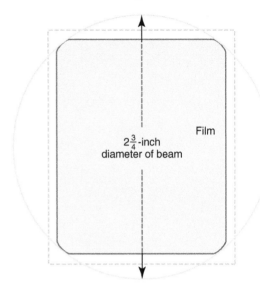

Film

$2\frac{3}{4}$-inch
diameter of beam

3. (Figure 2-3) Explain how this diagram of alternating current shows the effect of dental x-rays.

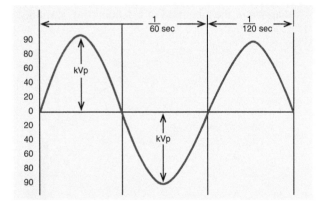

_____

_____

_____

4. (Figure 2-4) Indicate where characteristic x-rays are shown on this diagram.

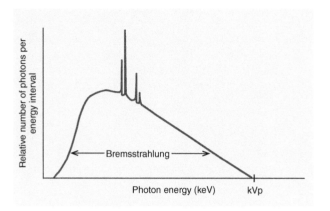

5. (Figure 2-5) What is the remedy for the condition illustrated on this diagram?

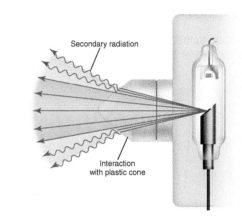

_____

_____

_____

CHAPTER 3

Image Formation

1. (Figure 3-1) Which tube head (used to produce the same image) will result in greater radiation exposure to the patient, A or B? Or would the patient receive the same amount of radiation exposure with either one?

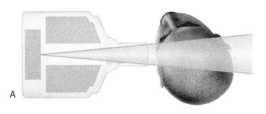

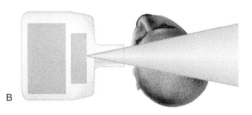

_____

_____

_____

_____

2. (Figure 3-2) If the exposure time for position A of the focal area is 20 impulses at 65 kVp and 10 mA, what would the exposure time be at position B, with the same kVp and mA, to produce the same radiograph?

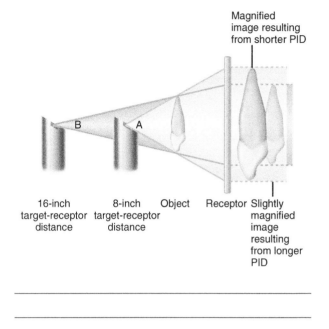

_____

_____

_____

3. (Figure 3-3) In this diagram of the bisecting technique, how would you describe the image that is produced?

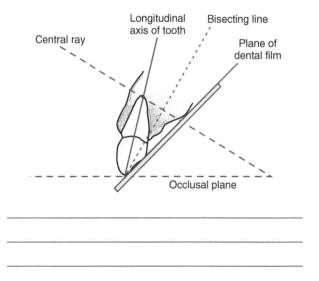

_____

_____

_____

181

4. (Figure 3-4) Label the target-receptor distance, object-receptor distance, and the focal-object distance.

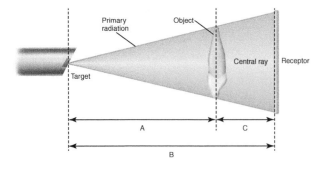

a.

b.

c.

5. (Figure 3-5) In this five-step density scale, between which areas is there the greatest contrast? Which areas have the least contrast?

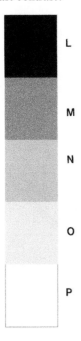

_____

_____

_____

CHAPTER 4

Image Receptors

1. (Figure 4-1) In this H and D curve, explain which receptor, A or B, would give the patient the least amount of radiation exposure.

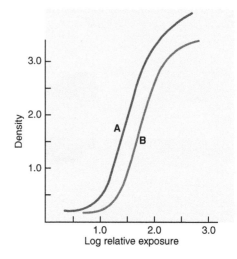

_____

_____

_____

2. (Figure 4-2) Label the film packets with their appropriate film size.

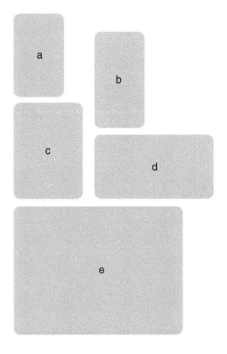

a. _____

b. _____

c. _____

d. _____

e. _____

3. (Figure 4-3) Label (A to F) the components of the intraoral film packet and explain each of their functions.

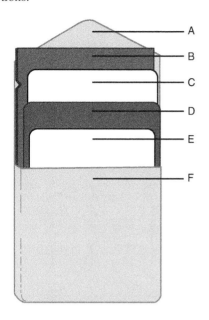

a. _____

_____

b. _____

_____

c. _____

_____

d. _____

_____

e. _____

_____

f. _____

_____

4. (Figure 4-4) What is the difference in exposure times between A and B? Explain.

A

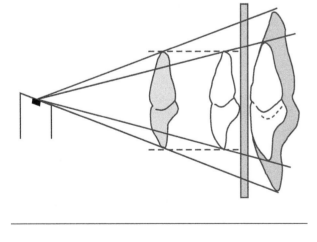

B

_____

_____

_____

5. (Figure 4-5) What is the relationship between object-receptor distance (OFD) and image magnification as depicted below?

_____

_____

_____

_____

CHAPTER 5

Biologic Effects of Radiation

1. Draw and label a nonthreshold dose-response curve.

2. Illustrate the Compton effect of x-ray interaction.

3. Draw a patient's face and illustrate primary and secondary radiation (as found in Chapter 6 of the textbook).

4. Illustrate the difference between localized and total body exposure on a figure of a seated patient.

5. Draw a threshold dose-response curve.

CHAPTER 6

Patient Protection

1. Draw the different relationships of the x-ray beam and secondary radiation to the thyroid gland using both the paralleling and bisecting techniques.

2. Illustrate how less tissue volume is exposed using a 16-inch target-receptor distance (FFD) rather than an 8-inch target-receptor distance (FFD).

Operator Protection

1. Draw a diagram of a dental operatory and indicate where the operator should stand when taking a radiographic exposure.

2. Draw a diagram identifying the areas of minimum and maximum scatter during dental x-ray exposure.

Infection Control in Dental Radiography

Identify the errors illustrated in Figures 8-1 through 8-5.

1. (Figure 8-1)

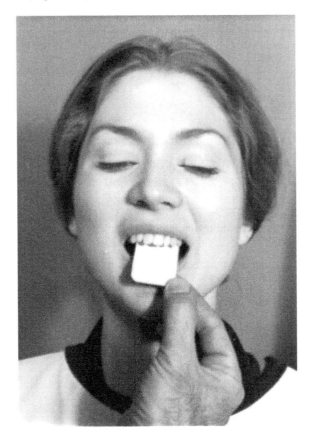

_____

_____

_____

2. (Figure 8-2)

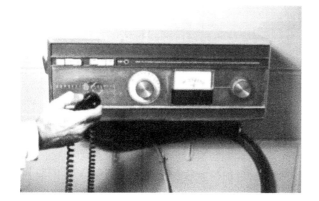

_____

_____

_____

3. (Figure 8-3)

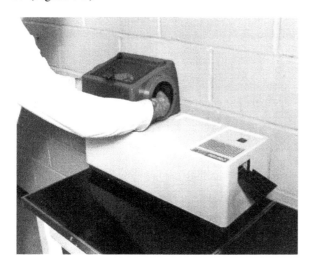

_____

_____

_____

4. (Figure 8-4)

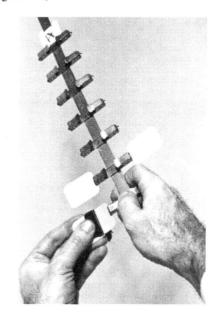

_____

_____

_____

5. (Figure 8-5)

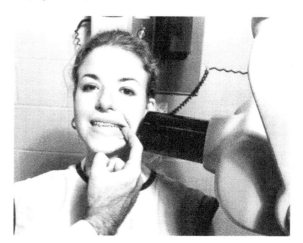

_____

_____

_____

CHAPTER 9

Intraoral Radiographic Technique: The Paralleling Method

1. (Figure 9-1) What error is illustrated here? How would you correct it?

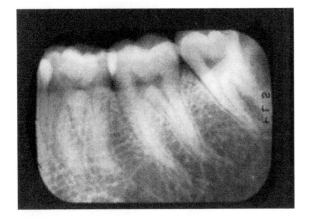

_____

_____

_____

2. (Figure 9-2) What error is illustrated here? How would you correct it?

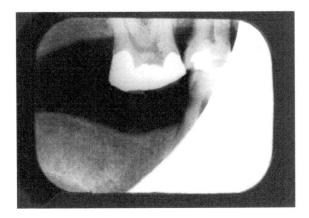

_____

_____

_____

3. (Figure 9-3) What error is illustrated here? How would you correct it?

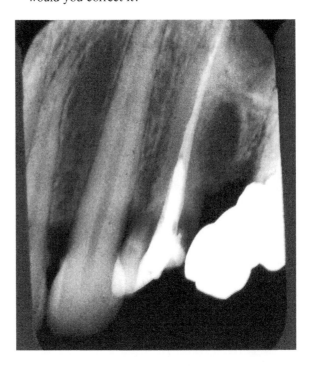

_____

_____

_____

4. (Figure 9-4) What error is illustrated here? What would you do to prevent its repetition?

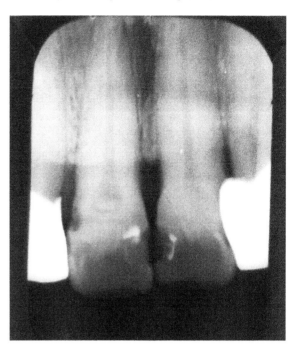

_____

_____

_____

5. (Figure 9-5) What error is illustrated here? What would you do to prevent its repetition?

_____

_____

_____

6. (Figure 9-6) What error is illustrated here? What are the possible causes for this error?

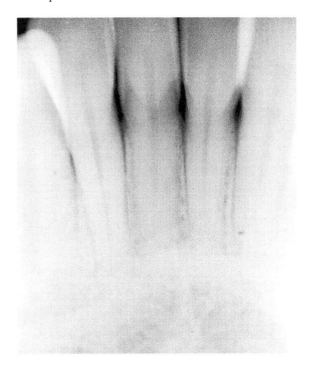

_____

_____

_____

7. (Figure 9-7) What chairside error could result in the following image? What is the remedy for this error?

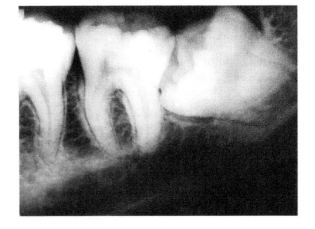

_____

_____

_____

CHAPTER 10

Accessory Radiographic Techniques: Bisecting Technique and Occlusal Projections

1. Draw the correct relationship of the central ray, teeth, and receptor in a diagram of horizontal angulation using the bisecting technique as compared with the paralleling technique.

2. Diagram the relationship of the central ray, tooth, and receptor for the bisecting technique.

3. (Figure 10-1) Which of these maxillary molar periapical projections, A or B, was taken with the paralleling technique? Which was taken with the bisecting technique? How did you determine your answer? Explain.

A

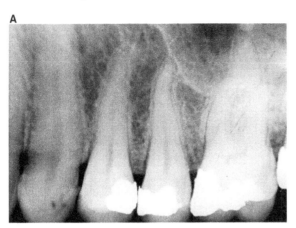

B

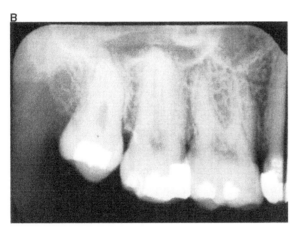

_____

_____

_____

_____

_____

4. (Figure 10-2) What error was made here? What caused it?

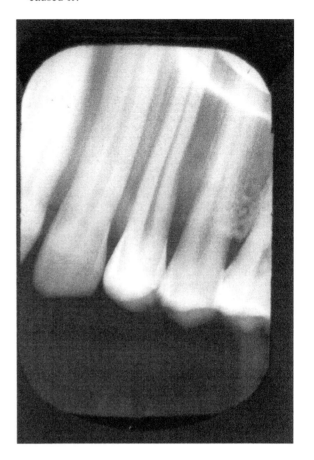

_____

_____

_____

5. (Figure 10-3) Was too little or too much vertical angulation used to produce this radiograph? What error is the result?

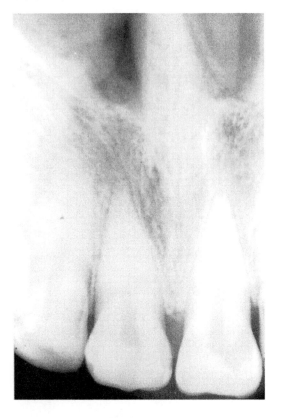

_____

_____

_____

6. (Figure 10-4) Identify the error seen here, and explain how you would correct it.

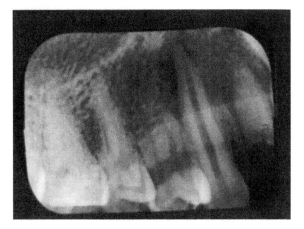

_____

_____

_____

7. (Figure 10-5) In this image taken with the bisecting technique, how would you describe the image? What technique error caused it?

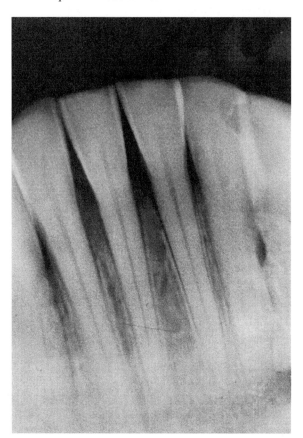

_____

_____

_____

CHAPTER 11

Film Processing Techniques

1. (Figure 11-1) What stages of the developing process are seen diagrammatically in this figure (1, 2, 3 and 4)?

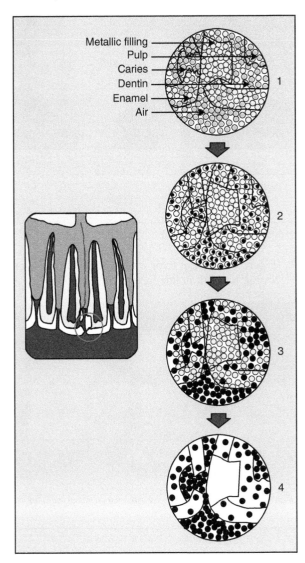

1. _____

2. _____

3. _____

4. _____

2. (Figure 11-2) List the possible cause for the film fog seen in this figure. What is the implication of the evidence shown in figure B?

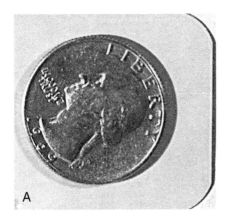

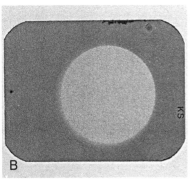

_____

_____

_____

3. (Figure 11-3) Identify the error seen in this figure. What is the cause of this error?

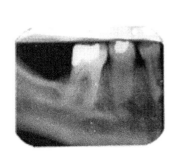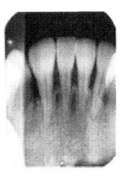

_____

_____

_____

4. (Figure 11-4) Name three possible causes that could produce a film like that seen in this figure.

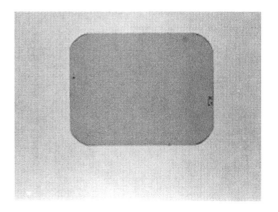

_____

_____

_____

5. (Figure 11-5) What could cause the error seen in this figure?

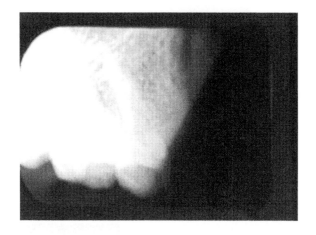

_____

_____

_____

6. (Figure 11-6) What error results in the artifacts seen in this figure?

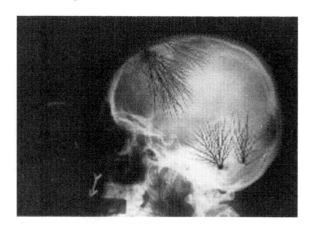

_____

_____

_____

7. (Figure 11-7) What error was made in automatic processing to result in this figure?

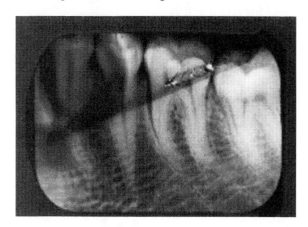

_____

_____

_____

8. (Figure 11-8) What error produces the processing error seen in this figure?

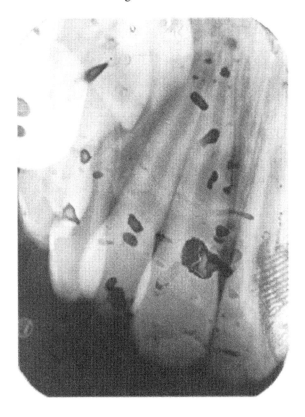

_____

_____

_____

9. (Figure 11-9) What error can produce a radiograph such as the one in this figure?

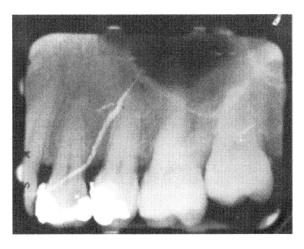

_____

_____

_____

10. (Figure 11-10) Interpret the result of the safelight (coin) test shown in this figure.

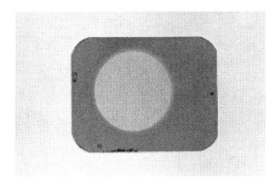

_____

_____

_____

CHAPTER 12

Panoramic Radiography

1. (Figure 12-1) What error is shown here?

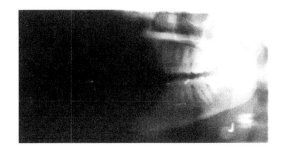

_____

_____

_____

2. (Figure 12-2) What error was produced here?

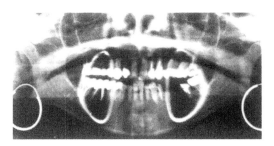

_____

_____

_____

3. (Figure 12-3) What error was produced here?

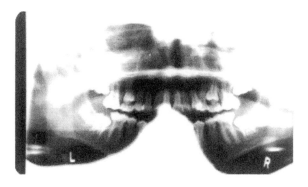

_____

_____

_____

4. (Figure 12-4) What error was produced here?

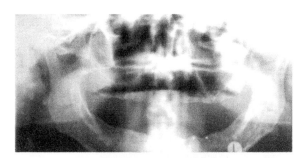

_____

_____

_____

5. (Figure 12-5) What error was produced here?

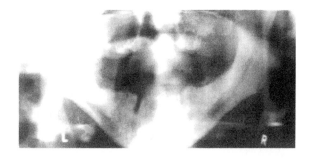

_____

_____

_____

6. (Figure 12-6) What is the circular radiopaque structure in the right posterior maxilla?

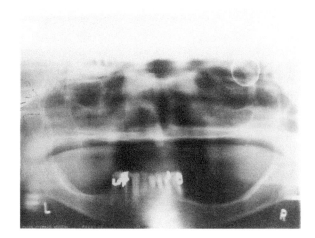

_____

_____

_____

CHAPTER 13

Extraoral Techniques

1. (Figure 13-1) Identify this radiographic projection.

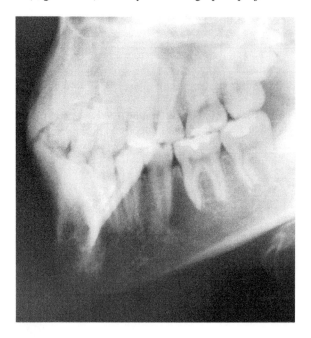

_____

_____

_____

2. Draw a schematic of the radiographic technique used for the projection in Figure 13-1.

4. Draw a schematic of the radiographic technique used for the projection in Figure 13-2.

3. (Figure 13-2) Identify this radiographic projection.

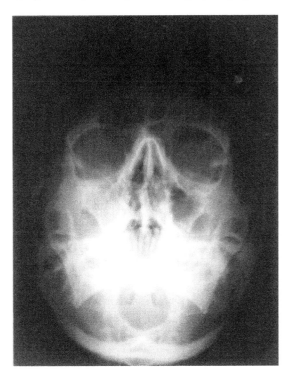

_____

_____

_____

5. (Figure 13-3) Identify this radiographic projection.

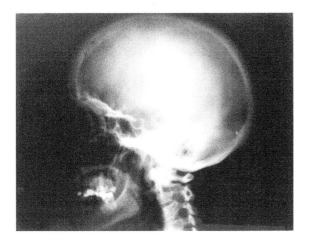

_____

_____

_____

197

6. Draw a schematic of the radiographic technique used for the projection in Figure 13-3.

8. (Figure 13-4) Identify this radiographic projection.

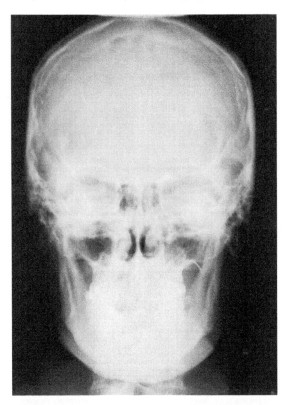

_____

_____

_____

7. Make a drawing that illustrates the use of a grid in dental radiography.

9. (Figure 13-5) What radiographic projection is seen here? Be specific!

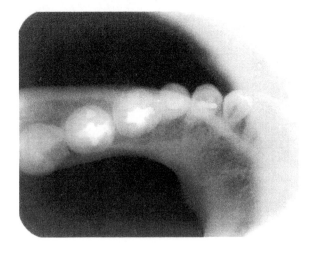

_____

_____

_____

10. (Figure 13-6) What radiographic projection is seen here? Be specific!

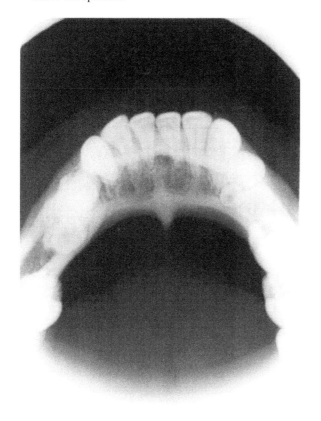

_____

_____

_____

CHAPTER 14

Radiography of the Temporomandibular Joint

1. Draw a diagram of the normal temporomandibular joint and label all of the essential components.

2. (Figure 14-1) Identify all of the essential components in the tomogram of the TMJ. Draw a line to the structure and label it accordingly.

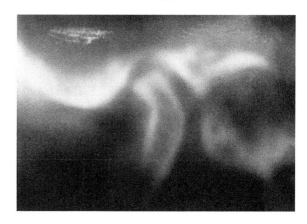

CHAPTER 15

Digital Imaging

1. (Figure 15-1) Can the following error occur with digital radiography? Explain.

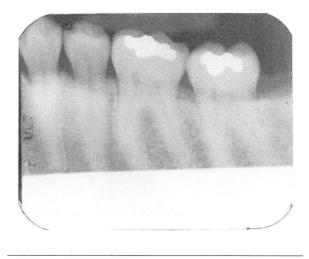

_____

_____

_____

_____

2. (Figure 15-2) Can the following error occur with digital radiography? Explain.

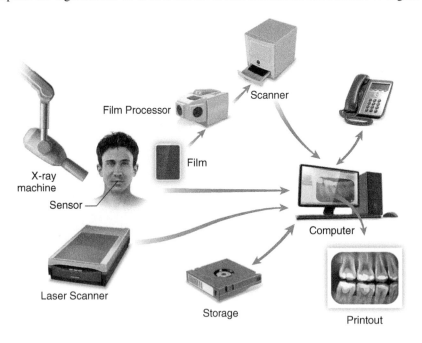

_____

_____

_____

3. (Figure 15-3) What does this photo represent?

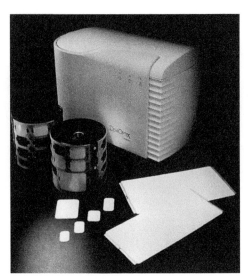

_____

_____

_____

4. (Figure 15-4) Explain the significance of what is shown in this illustration in reference to digital radiography.

X-ray machine
Sensor
Film Processor
Film
Scanner
Laser Scanner
Storage
Computer
Printout

_____

_____

_____

_____

_____

CHAPTER 16

Advanced Imaging Systems

1. (Figure 16-1) What advanced imaging system is displayed in the following illustration? What is the source of energy used to capture the image? What is being used as the receptor in this technique?

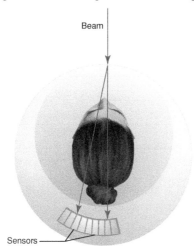

Beam

Sensors

_____

_____

_____

_____

_____

2. (Figure 16-2) What is the illustration below exhibiting? What is the significance of this information in dental CT and CBCT scanning?

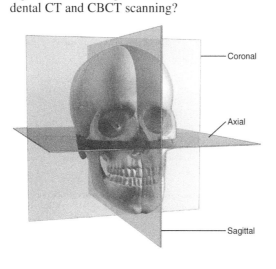

Coronal

Axial

Sagittal

_____

_____

_____

_____

3. (Figure 16-3) What technique was utilized to capture the following image? Which "window" is being displayed?

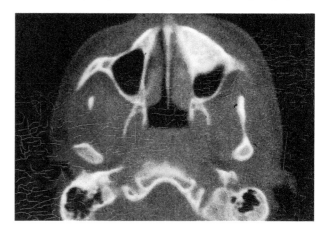

_____

_____

_____

4. (Figure 16-4) What technique was utilized to capture the following image? Which "window" is being displayed?

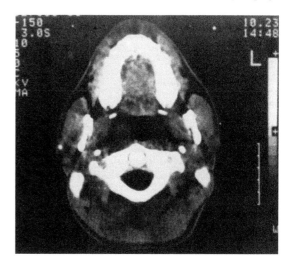

_____

_____

_____

201

5. (Figure 16-5) What advanced imaging technique was used to capture this image? What do the white areas represent? What do the dark areas represent? What is the most common use for this imaging technique in dentistry?

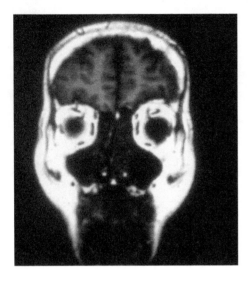

_____

_____

_____

_____

CHAPTER 17

Quality Assurance

1. (Figure 17-1) What test for quality assurance in the darkroom is pictured below? What does it test for? What does the procedure involved consist of?

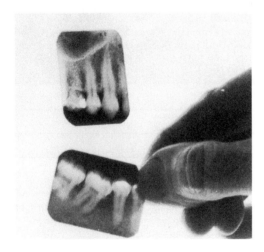

_____

_____

_____

2. (Figure 17-2) What test for quality assurance in the darkroom is pictured below? What does it test for? What does the procedure involved consist of?

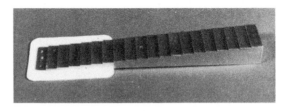

_____

_____

_____

_____

3. (Figure 17-3) What is shown in the illustration below? What is it used for?

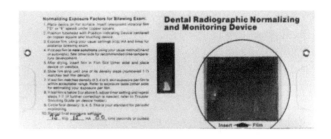

_____

_____

_____

4. (Figure 17-4) What procedure is this illustration showing? Explain.

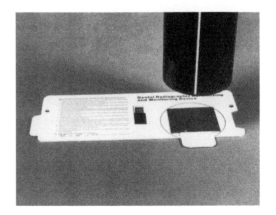

_____

_____

_____

5. (Figure 17-5) What procedure is shown in the following illustration? Explain.

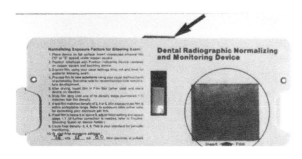

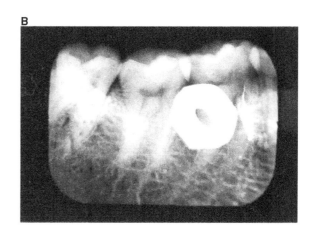

_____

_____

_____

CHAPTER 18

Patient Management and Special Problems

1. (Figure 18-1) Radiograph B was taken with an increased distal horizontal angulation from the initial radiograph A. Thus the foreign body must be:
   a. located buccally
   b. located lingually
   c. in a location that cannot be determined

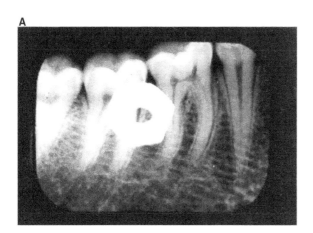

2. (Figure 18-2) What type of radiograph is this? What would be its use?

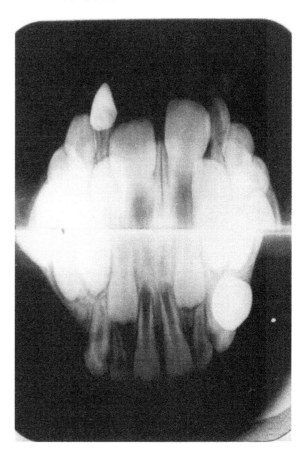

_____

_____

_____

_____

203

CHAPTER 19

Film Mounting and Radiographic Anatomy

Identify the lettered structures on each of the following radiographs.

1. (Figure 19-1) Identify the labeled structures.

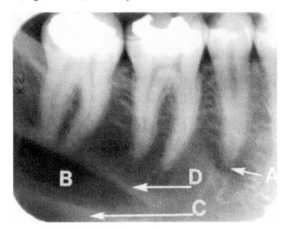

a. _____

b. _____

c. _____

d. _____

2. (Figure 19-2) Which intraoral radiographic projection is this? Assuming labial mounting, which side of the mouth is this? Identify the labeled structures.

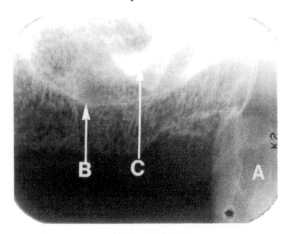

_____

_____

a. _____

b. _____

c. _____

3. (Figure 19-3) Identify the following structures labeled A through F.

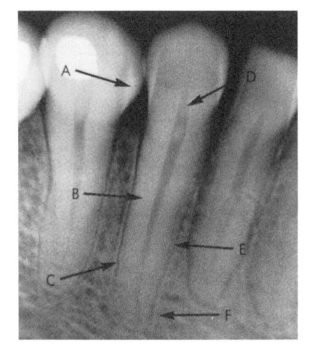

a. _____

b. _____

c. _____

d. _____

e. _____

f. _____

4. (Figure 19-4) Which intraoral radiographic projection is this? Identify the labeled structures.

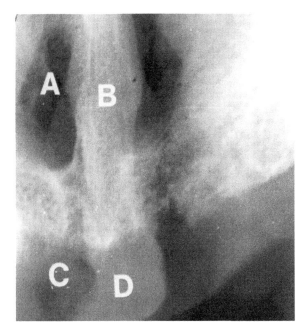

_____

a. _____

b. _____

c. _____

d. _____

5. (Figure 19-5) Identify the labeled structures.

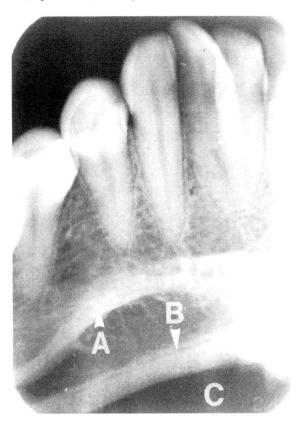

a. _____

b. _____

c. _____

6. (Figure 19-6) Identify structures A and B.

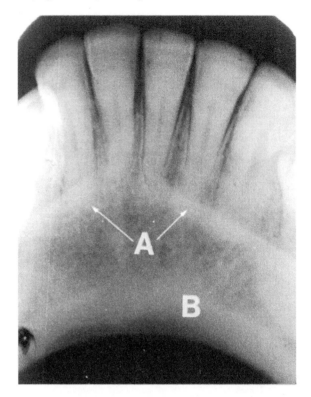

a. _____

b. _____

7. (Figure 19-7) Identify the labeled structures.

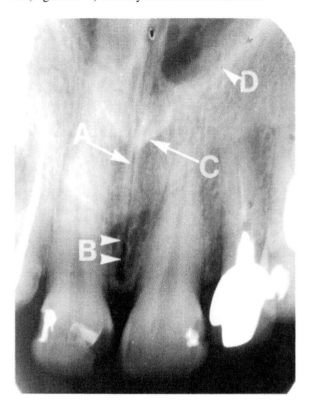

a. _____

b. _____

c. _____

d. _____

8. (Figure 19-8) Identify the labeled structures.

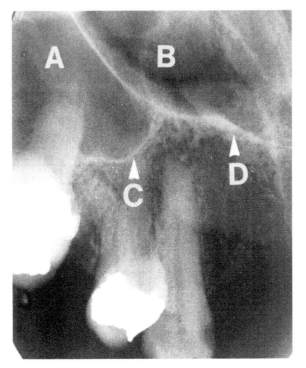

a. _____

b. _____

c. _____

d. _____

9. (Figure 19-9) Identify A and B.

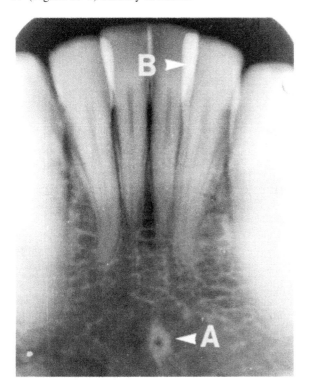

a. _____

b. _____

10. (Figure 19-10) Identify A and B.

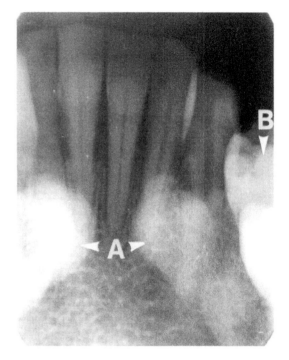

a. _____

b. _____

11. (Figure 19-11) What radiographic view is this? Assuming labial mounting, is it the patient's right or left? Identify the labeled structures.

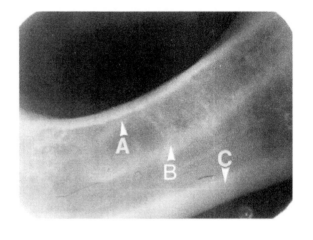

_____

_____

a. _____

b. _____

c. _____

12. (Figure 19-12) Identify the labeled structures.

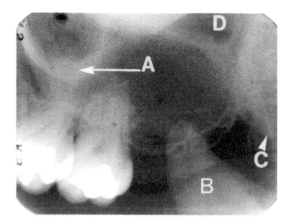

a. _____

b. _____

c. _____

d. _____

13. (Figure 19-13) Identify the labeled structures.

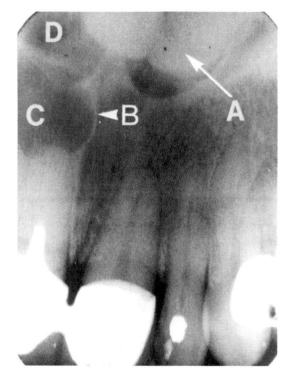

a. _____

b. _____

c. _____

d. _____

14. (Figure 19-14) Identify A and B.

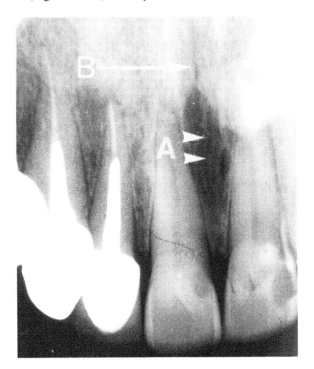

a. _____

b. _____

15. (Figure 19-15) All teeth test vital. What is your interpretation of the radiolucency at the apex of the second premolar?

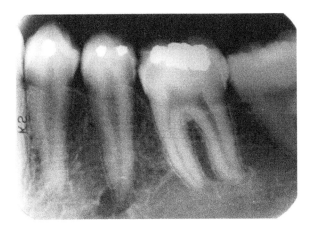

_____

_____

_____

16. (Figure 19-16) Assuming labial mounting, what side (left or right) and area does this radiograph show? Identify the labeled structures.

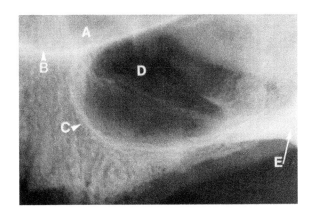

a. _____

b. _____

c. _____

d. _____

e. _____

17. (Figure 19-17) Identify the radiopaque dense bony structure seen at the top of this radiograph.

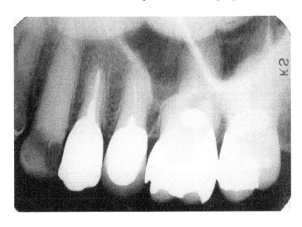

_____

_____

_____

18. (Figure 19-18) Identify the radiopaque dense area of bone outlined by the arrows.

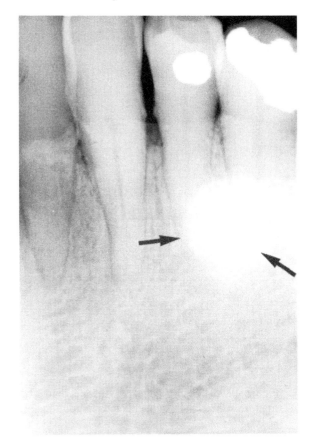

_____

_____

_____

CHAPTER 20

Principles of Radiographic Interpretation

1. (Figure 20-1) What type of radiographic image is this? Describe the status of tooth #18. Explain.

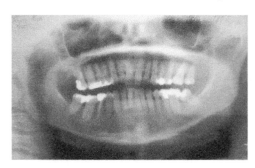

_____

_____

_____

2. (Figure 20-2) What is the possible identification of the lesion? What is its effect on the surrounding structures?

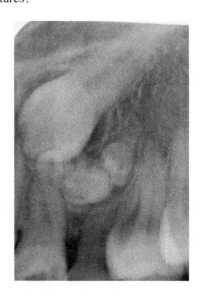

_____

_____

_____

3. (Figure 20-3) Describe the lesion below. Include the location of the lesion and whether it is an RL, RO, or mixed lesion. What is the possible identification of the lesion?

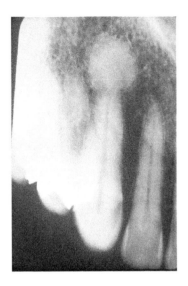

_____

_____

_____

4. (Figure 20-4) Identify which of the following lesions in the image below is normal anatomy and which is a cyst (the lesion toward the patient's right or the lesion toward the patient's left). Explain how you came to this conclusion.

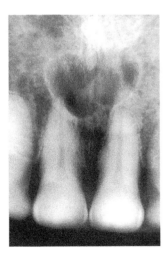

_____

_____

_____

_____

5. (Figure 20-5) Describe the lesion near the root of tooth #29. Include the location of the lesion and whether it is an RL, RO, or mixed lesion. What is the possible identification of the lesion? Is it a pathology or normal anatomy?

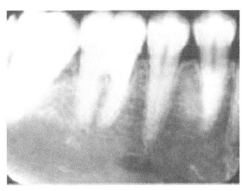

_____

_____

_____

_____

_____

CHAPTER 21

Caries and Periodontal Disease

1. (Figure 21-1) Identify the caries on this radiograph.

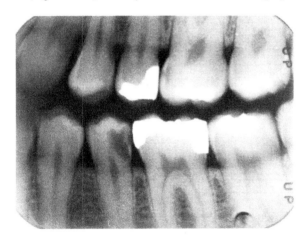

_____

_____

_____

2. (Figure 21-2) Identify the caries on this radiograph.

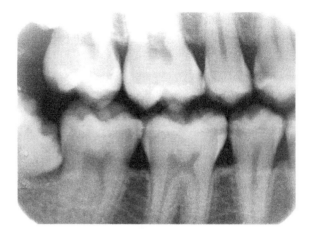

_____

_____

_____

4. (Figure 21-4) What periodontal conditions appear on this radiograph?

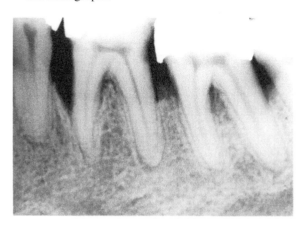

_____

_____

_____

3. (Figure 21-3) How would you classify the periodontal bone conditions on this radiograph?

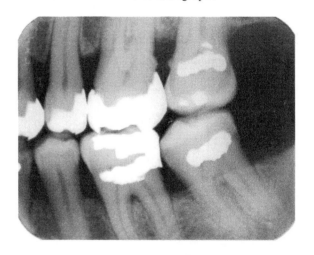

_____

_____

_____

5. (Figure 21-5) Differentiate between the cervical radiolucencies seen on the mesial and distal surfaces of the first molar. How would you confirm your radiographic interpretation?

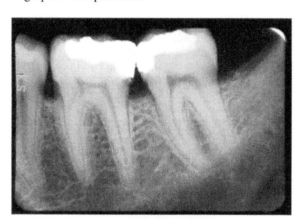

_____

_____

_____

6. (Figure 21-6) What is your interpretation of the radiolucent area seen on the mesial of the canine?

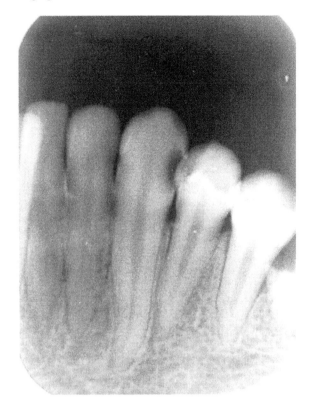

7. (Figure 21-7) Identify the caries, if any, on this radiograph.

_____

_____

_____

_____

_____

_____

8. (Figure 21-8) What type of periodontal bone change appears on this radiograph?

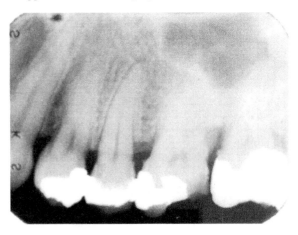

_____

_____

_____

9. (Figure 21-9) Locate the calculus on this radiograph.

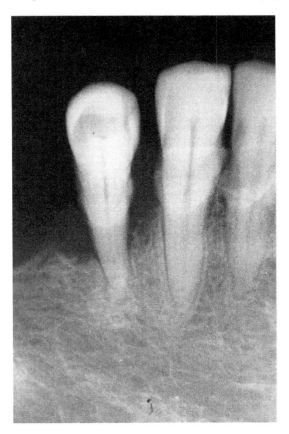

_____

_____

_____

10. (Figure 21-10) Locate the caries on this radiograph.

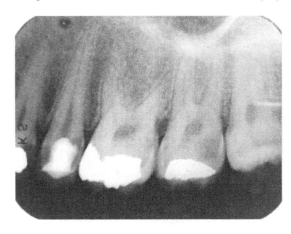

_____

_____

_____

11. (Figure 21-11) How would you classify the periodontal condition shown here? What is the prognosis?

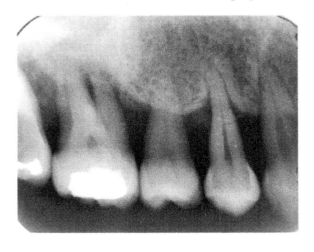

_____

_____

_____

12. (Figure 21-12) Identify the caries in this radiograph.

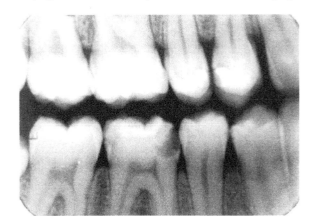

_____

_____

_____

13. (Figure 21-13) Identify the radiopaque area pointed out by the arrow.

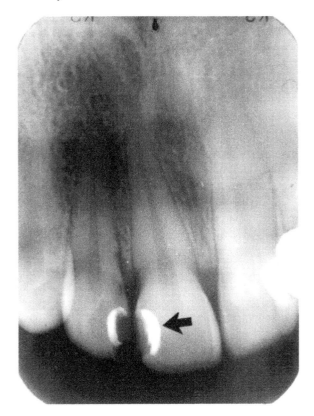

_____

_____

_____

CHAPTER 22

Pulpal and Periapical Lesions

1. (Figure 22-1) There is pain and tenderness in the mucobuccal fold in the area of the extracted central incisor. All teeth test vital. What is your possible interpretation of this radiolucent area?

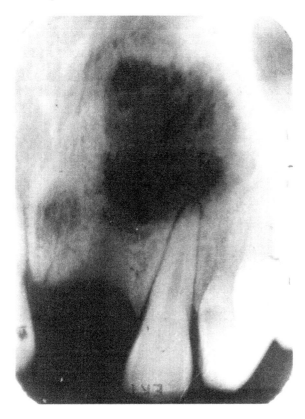

_____

_____

_____

2. (Figure 22-2) This radiograph was taken of an asymptomatic new patient. What is your possible interpretation for the condition seen here?

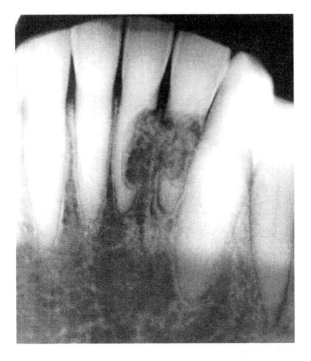

_____

_____

_____

3. (Figure 22-3) What is your interpretation of this condition seen in this 49-year-old woman where all teeth test vital?

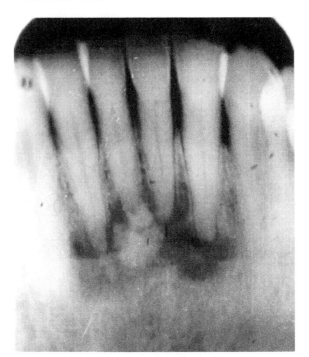

_____

_____

_____

4. (Figure 22-4) The lower first molar is nonvital. What is your possible interpretation of the radiopacity on the distal root?

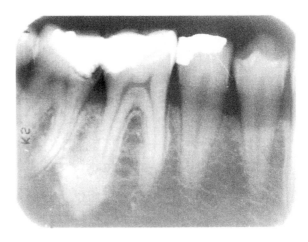

_____

_____

_____

5. (Figure 22-5) Pain and swelling are associated with the lateral incisor. What is your possible interpretation?

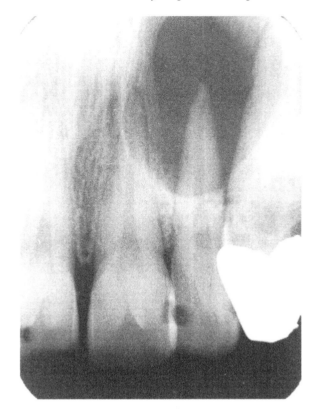

_____

_____

_____

6. (Figure 22-6) Identify the radiolucent areas A and B. Note the incomplete endodontic filling in the first premolar.

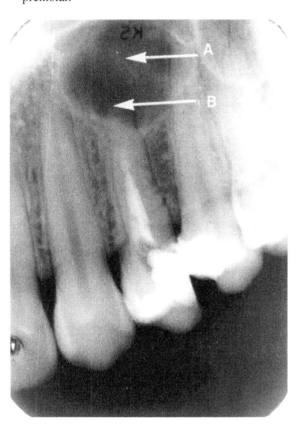

a. _____

b. _____

Developmental Disturbances of Teeth and Bone

Identify the following tooth conditions.

1. (Figure 23-1).

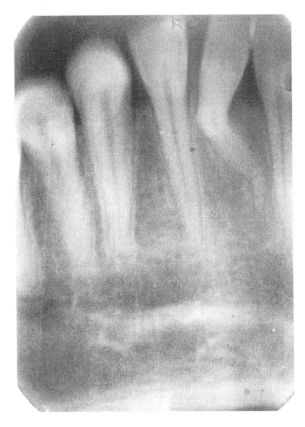

_____

_____

_____

2 (Figure 23-2).

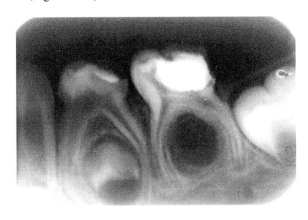

_____

_____

_____

3. (Figure 23-3).

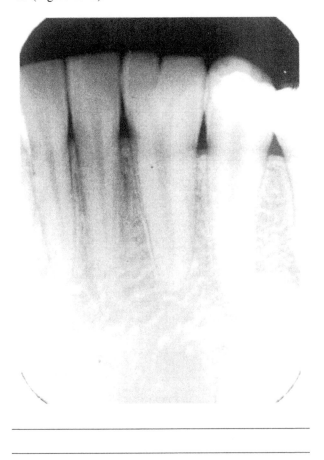

_____

_____

_____

4. (Figure 23-4).

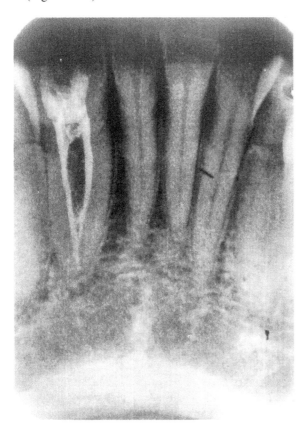

_____
_____
_____

5. (Figure 23-5).

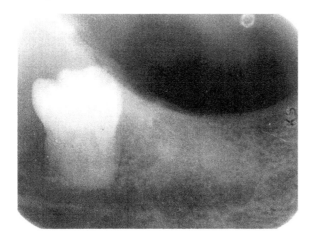

_____
_____
_____

CHAPTER 24

Bone and Other Lesions

Identify the following tooth conditions.

1. (Figure 24-1) What is your possible interpretation of the conditions seen on this panoramic radiograph?

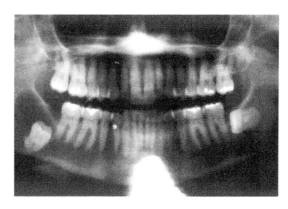

_____
_____
_____

2. (Figure 24-2) What is your possible interpretation of the tumor shown here?

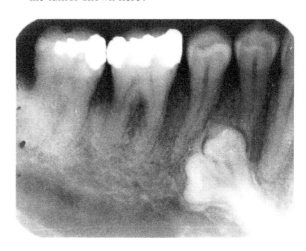

_____
_____
_____

3. (Figure 24-3) What is your interpretation of the radiopaque structure seen here?

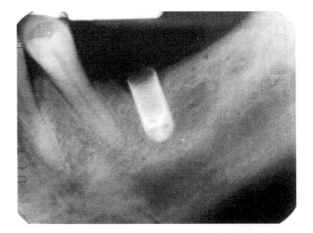

_____

_____

_____

4. (Figure 24-4) This patient fell off a bicycle, sustaining lacerations to the lip and cheek. The canine is extremely painful to touch. What is your possible interpretation?

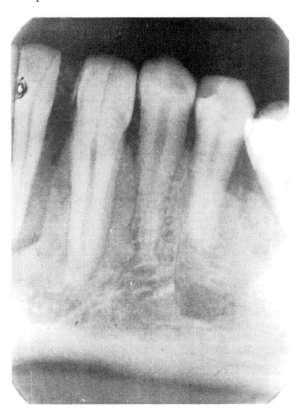

_____

_____

_____

5. (Figure 24-5) Give two possible interpretations of the radiopaque area the arrows are pointing to in this illustration.

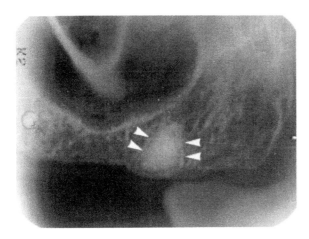

_____

_____

_____